Souls on a Walk:

An Enduring Love Story
Unbroken By Alzheimer's

by John Geyman

"*Souls on a Walk* traces the clinical progression of the disease with a human voice giving the reader the opportunity to place himself into the story and ask 'how would I be able to handle either role?' Both were a caregiver to the other by reason of early recognition then diagnosis, i.e. before the disease took complete control of both lives. I read the book straight through, and could not put it down."

—Ed Greub, Friday Harbor, WA

"Brains don't get Alzheimer's disease; people get Alzheimer's disease. John Geyman utilizes his observational skills honed over decades as a family physician to present a compelling account of his wife Gene and how the disease affected both of them. Love shines through from every page."

–Howard Brody, M.D., Ph.D., Director of the Institute for the Medical Humanities at the University of Texas Medical Branch in Galveston and author of *Stories of Sickness*

"What a privilege to read *Souls on a Walk*. I was surprised by the powerful pull of the story—every reader knows the ending, at least its broad outlines, yet it was an emotional page-turner."

—Greg Bates, president and publisher of Common Courage Press, Monroe, Maine

Souls on a Walk - An Enduring Love Story
Unbroken By Alzheimers

Cover photo by Floris van Breugel
Interior and cover design by W. Bruce Conway

This is a work of non-fiction.
All characters and events portrayed in this book are true

ISBN: 978-0-9837734-5-0

Edited by Emily Reed
Published by Copernicus Healthcare
Distributed by: LightningSource/Ingram
Printed in the United States of America

Copernicus Healthcare is donating 10% of each sale of this
book to help fund Alzheimer's research and support programs. To learn more about Alzheimer's disease,
go to: www. alz.org

Souls on a Walk:

**An Enduring Love Story
Unbroken By Alzheimer's**

Dedication

To Gene: The Love and Light of My Life Forever,
Wherever We Are...

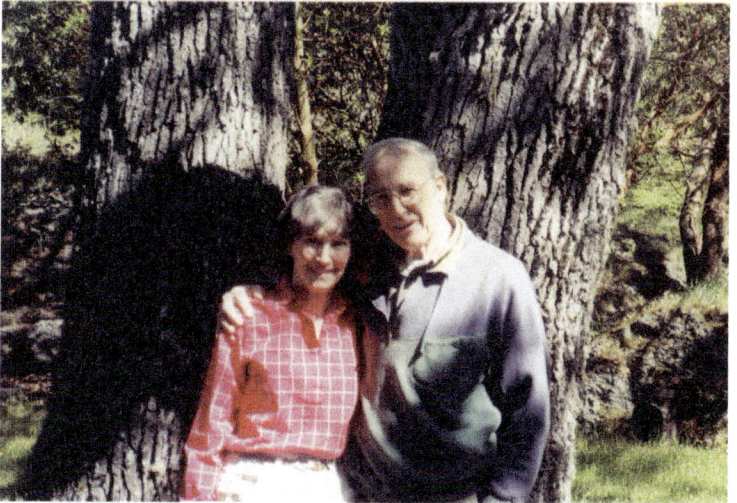

SOUL ON A WALK

I took my soul out for a walk one time
drenched it in sunset beauty
submerged it in the peaceful quiet
of calm and passive twilight
then let it rest
serene upon a bed of midnight blue
under a stream of calm moonlight
until, all pure and lovely,
it was roused by pulsing stars.
I took my soul out
for a walk one time
and oh, the change.

—Gene Geyman,

Late 1950s

CONTENTS

PART III

TOWARD A NEW FUTURE

PREFACE

I have debated with myself whether or not to write this book.

There were many reasons why I should not. There are already other books by caregivers who have gone through this hellish journey in dealing with Alzheimer's. I don't like to write about myself. To do so in a first-person voice is not my style of writing, and bares a raw soul if I am to keep this story completely honest, as I must.

There are still other reasons not to write the story of one couple's dealing with Alzheimer's. This disease is highly variable, whether by age of onset, how it progresses, or its impacts on patients and family members. As they say, tell me about one case of Alzheimer's and you know about just that one.

Despite these reasons, I am going to tell this story for other reasons. First, in tribute to Gene, a magnificent person who showed such courage and grace in triumphing over the ravages of this disease in her own special way. And to give thanks to her for making me the luckiest man in the world for having shared our lives together over all these years. I am necessarily part of Gene's story, for this is really *our* story over 56 years of a marriage blessed in heaven.

In order to better understand how the disease affected us, I will share some highlights before the onset of her Alzheimer's at age 61, and how the disease changed our lives over the next 16 years. I was the caregiver over all those years. She was at home all the way until the last five days, and even then I was with her in her hospital room, and finally in her hospice room.

So, whether I like it or not, this book necessarily shares raw feelings of a long-term painful experience punctuated by many spectacular breakthroughs of her buoyant spirit that still leave me in awe of her character and special grace. Each of us has our own narrative that we bring to how we will respond to the challenges of this kind of disease. In this situation, I will try to point out instances that had everything to do with how Gene dealt with her own Alzheimer's.

Another reason to write this book is to hope that this story, though just one of hundreds of thousands playing out every day among families so afflicted, will be useful to others having to deal with this disease, soon to become the second leading cause of death in America as our population ages. So many patients and caregivers deal with this illness (which becomes a *family* illness) in isolation without much sharing with others. And yes, Alzheimer's affects every patient in different ways, but there are still many commonalities for those of us navigating our ways through it. Here I will try to point out some of the bigger challenges, and how Gene and I together coped with them. And as any reader will already gather, writing this book is therapy for me. It is a search for meaning in helping me to better understand what has happened, and being able to move on with my next chapter.

Since Gene died, I have heard varied accounts of how others, men and women, have managed after death of their spouses in long happy marriages. Each responded to their enormous losses in their own particular ways. One grieving husband bought a new RV, put his wife's name on a second license plate, and planned to travel "together" to many of their favorite places around the country. Here, I will stay at home, surrounded by pictures and Gene's spirit, and recall many of our special memories over 56 years as a means to better appreciate the meaning of our lives together.

You can imagine the difficulty of summarizing and portraying this story over most of two lifetimes. How to organize this book? I have chosen to break it into three parts, mostly chronological. In order to give you a picture of Gene's character and personality and to understand how they were impacted by her disease. I will intersperse her own words at times to give you a better understanding of Gene, the person. Part I deals with our lives before the onset of Alzheimer's. Part II highlights our 16-year journey with the disease; within that I will try to intersperse both of our concerns and feelings as her disease progressed, including some humorous vignettes that broke through our pain. Part III will deal with my reflections in bereavement, what I have learned, and going forward with my next chapter.

This will be our personal journey before, during and after Alzheimer's. Come along and let me share with you the courage, resilience and grace of Gene, a remarkable human being, with whom I had the good fortune to spend most of my life. So here goes, often through my tears, but your paper will be dry!

PART I

*From Courtship in 1955 to
Alzheimer's in 1996*

Chapter 1

How We Met

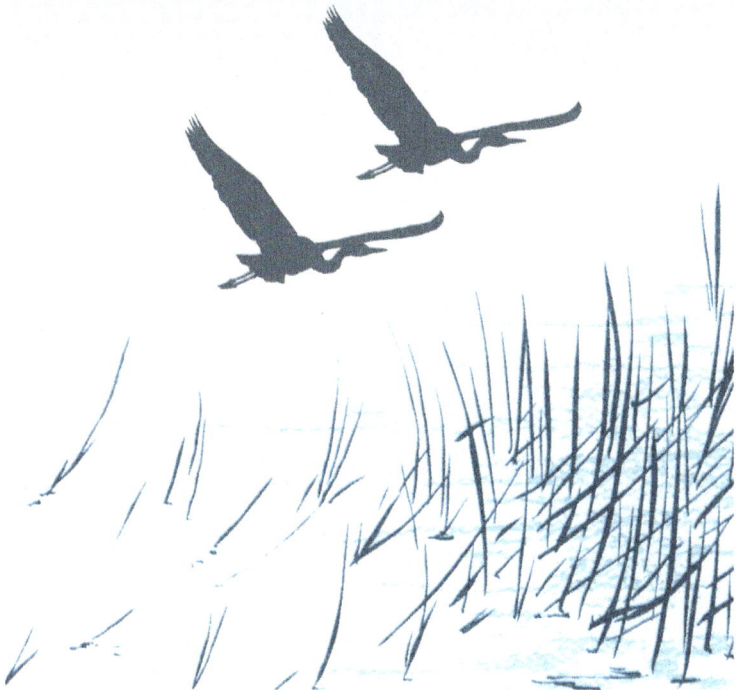

It was love at first sight. Here's what happened on a May day in Berkeley, California, in 1955. I was getting processed out of the Navy at Treasure Island after three years on a destroyer in the Pacific during and after the Korean War. So I called my sister Carolyn, then a junior at the University of California Berkeley, to see if she could arrange a blind double date for my friend Jim and me. She did so, putting me with a girl who had also gone East to college and Jim with Gene, her roommate in the Alpha Phi House. We went ice skating, and eight minutes into the date, we changed partners—for good! We skated away together the rest of the night and then talked until she nearly missed her curfew at the sorority. I can still remember what she was wearing—a beige blouse and a light green wool skirt.

Right off we found an amazing symmetry in our backgrounds, values and experiences. For starters, we had the same birthday—February 9th—though I was four years older. We both were optimists and open to life. We both enjoyed being with people. We both were readers and liked to talk about ideas. We both had been fortunate by birth in our families and backgrounds, though Gene had lost her dad in World War II.

From the start, we found that we could talk about anything and everything. She was smart, perky, funny, interesting and caring. She loved people and life. We dated for a year, then got married just after she graduated the following June.

I was the lucky one. When we met, she had four of-fers of marriage. One from a blind man to whom she had read through all four years of college, who later went on to marry and teach high school in Los Banos, California. Another to a future attorney, a third to a realtor, both in Marin County, and a fourth who earned a Ph.D. in History and joined the faculty at Columbia University.

During our courtship over that year, I finished up pre-medical requirements at Berkeley. Since I had gone through Princeton as a Geology major before the Navy years, I had most of the pre-med requirements still to do. During that year I lived off campus, did yard work for my board/room and hashed in another sorority.

We got engaged on our birthdays in February, then started planning for what to do after her graduation. I was accepted early on at the medical school at Washington University in St. Louis, but we wanted to stay west if pos-sible. Fortunately, the University of California San Fran-cisco accepted me, so that became our plan.

The first year of medical school at UCSF was still in Berkeley. It had been in San Francisco until the fire and earthquake of 1906, when the basic science build-ing was demolished. It was moved to Berkeley for the next 50 years, so that was where we spent the first year of our marriage. We found an apartment off campus to move into after our honeymoon.

The next thing, of course, was to furnish the apart-ment in advance. That included a bed. So we found a king bed, put it on the top of my Ford coupe, and drove it to our new apartment, both laughing in embarrassment. Rare today, we were both virgins.

We were married in the Episcopal church in Ross, California, on June 9, 1956. Though I had been much less of a churchgoer and closer to agnostic, she was kind enough to have this inscribed on my gold wedding ring: "Thy God Shall Be My God."

Our honeymoon was fun in surprising ways. Friends of my parents loaned us their cabin at Glenbrook on the Nevada side of Lake Tahoe for a week. A beautiful place, but we got bored there after two or three days. Gene had worked at Glacier Point in Yosemite for three summers during college, so why not go there for the rest of the week?

After negotiating the narrow and winding Tioga Pass road into Yosemite from the east, we arrived at Glacier Point Lodge, high above the Valley, in the midst of a storm. A cold front had moved in, and we were surrounded by clouds. Checking into the Lodge, we could only get a small austere room with steam heat that barely worked. There was nothing to do outside, and when we went out into the Lodge front area, Gene knew everyone from past summers. After two cold days in the clouds, we returned to Berkeley.

While I became immersed in gross anatomy, histology, biochemistry and such, Gene finished her practice teaching during that first year. She was a gifted and natural teacher from the start, giving so much to her kids. She taught the early primary grades over most of her teaching years. This picture shows how seriously she took teaching, but she could also laugh a lot along the way.

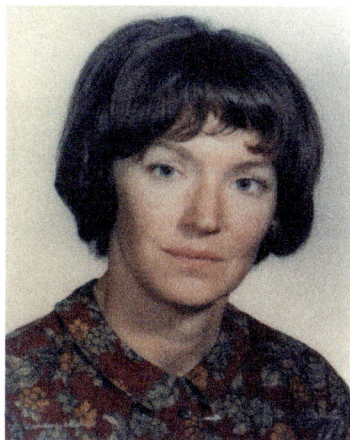

Chapter 2

Medical Education Years

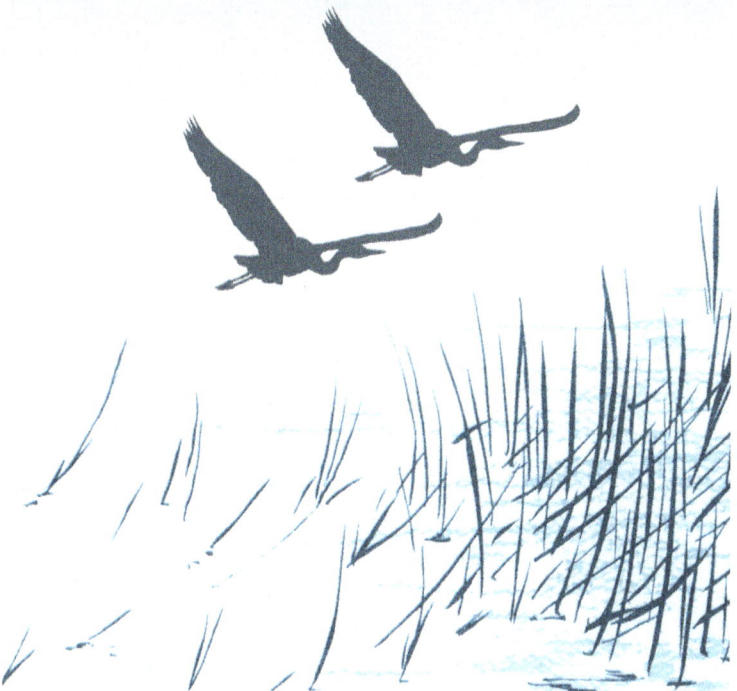

After our first year in Berkeley, we moved to a flat about a mile from the medical school in San Francisco. Gene was teaching full-time in South San Francisco, commuting daily. We had many good friends in my class, especially among those who had previously been in the service.

We counseled in a camp in Arizona during our second summer together. It was at the Orme School about 80 miles north of Phoenix, which also operates a camp for teenage kids every summer on its working cattle ranch. Gene taught riding and art, while I taught riflery, logical since I had been the Gunnery Officer on my destroyer. Since I had completed the first two years of medical school (and since we were 80 miles from a real doctor!), I was occasionally called upon to see a sick or injured camper. At that point I knew virtually no clinical medicine, but I'm glad they thought I did! We enjoyed the summer immensely, and even came to like the hot, barren high desert country.

Our first son, Matthew, was born in our junior year during a Thanksgiving visit to my parents in Santa Barbara. This started a pattern for Gene's future pregnancies. She was always interested in getting on with it sooner than later. Matt was born at 34 weeks after a rapid labor. I was in Los Angeles interviewing for internship at Los Angeles County General Hospital, sped up the freeway to Santa Barbara only to arrive five minutes late. Gene's later pregnancies ended just as quickly and successfully at 34 and 36 weeks. We didn't waste much time. All three of our sons were born within a three-year period!

After graduation from medical school in June of 1960, we went south to Los Angeles, settling in Temple City for the year while I did my internship at L.A. County, then the second largest hospital in the country with 3,500 beds. I thrived on all that, took extra rotations in obstetrics-gynecology (24 hours on, 24 off, with seven deliveries every shift) as well as general practice on the Jail Service, where we saw everything. Our second son, Cal, was born during that year, so Gene had her hands full.

Then we went north again the next year for two years of general practice residency training at Sonoma County Hospital in Santa Rosa, California. It was a busy county hospital with an excellent, well-established residency program. Ten of us residents ran the hospital with ready consultation and help from all the specialties in the community. We formed many lifelong friendships during those two years, and our third son, Sabin, was born during that time.

By the Fall of 1962 it was time to think about where we would go to practice when the residency ended the next June. We wanted a small community where we could make a difference. Gene was adaptable as always—she had moved 13 times in growing up in the South as her civil engineer dad moved with his crew during the Great Depression wherever there was work and as the family moved West after the outbreak of World War II. We wanted to find a small town somewhere in the Pacific Northwest, so we took a trip to look at Mt. Shasta, Hood River, OR, Anacortes and Pullman, WA, Moscow, ID, Whitefish and Kalispell in Montana. We almost went to Kalispell, even to the point of arranging for a small office to be built there just out of town on the Flathead River. But plans fell through when the contractor changed his mind. A good thing, since where the office would have been was washed away in a 1964 flood. And also good, we ended up in Mt. Shasta the next summer to start six great years in beautiful country closer to both of our families.

Chapter 3

Early Practice Years: Mt. Shasta

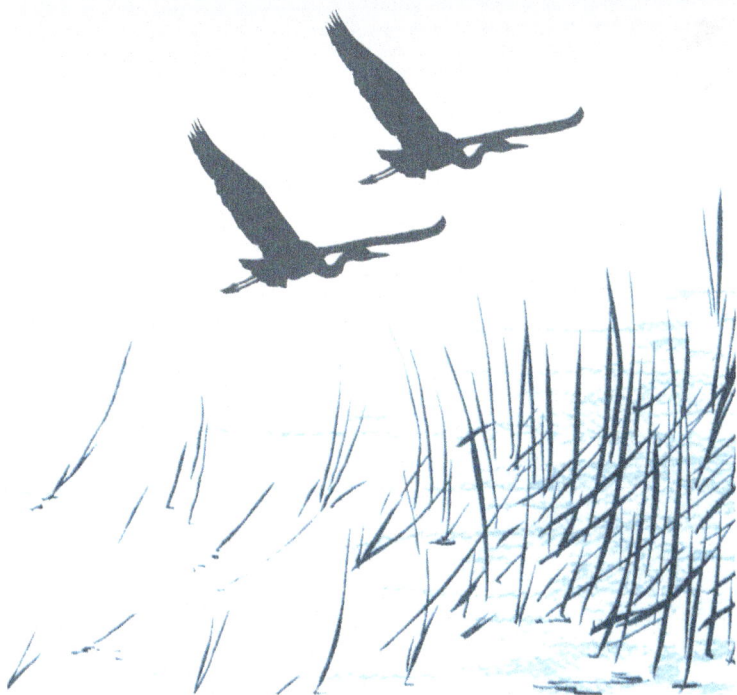

Our **Mt. Shasta years** were exhilarating and formative for both Gene and me. It was the first time for both of us to live in a small rural community. We both sought it out. A former railroad town (Southern Pacific Railroad), Mt. Shasta was still a logging town, originally settled by northern Italian loggers who found its country similar to the mountains of northern Italy. Great country, with Mount Shasta towering over the town at 14,161 feet.

We lived in town the first year, then found three acres three miles west of town on two streams and had a house built to our plans. We fenced an acre for Gene's horse and built a barn. Gene became fully involved with full-time teaching, working with the Cub scouts, teaching skiing, raising three active sons, and putting up with me.

I also thrived. We had a 28-bed hospital in town serving the three surrounding towns as well—Dunsmuir, Weed and McCloud. There were eight of us general practitioners/family physicians, all with several years of graduate training with practices ranging from internal medicine, pediatrics, obstetrics, trauma, and whatever common and urgent problems patients brought to us for care. Redding was our referral center to the south, Medford to the north. During that time we opened a coronary care unit in the hospital, the first in such a small hospital. There was no question that we were making a difference. More than 40 years later, I can still recall memories of house calls and situations in many of the houses in the area.

Here's a picture of Gene as a second-grade teacher

at Mt. Shasta Elementary School in 1968. Superintendent Isaac Kelsoe had successfully recruited Gene by persuading her that she was not busy enough with three kids under nine.

And here's a picture that shows another side of Gene, out in front of our new house with our three sons, with Mt. Shasta in the background.

Mt. Shasta was a diverse and friendly community, and we made many friends among the "locals" and others from out of town who built cabins in the area. Among those, Pat and John Thompson from Mill Valley in Marin County became lifelong friends. About ten years older than us and with four sons of their own, they built an A-frame cabin west of town for frequent family vacations. Just to give you a

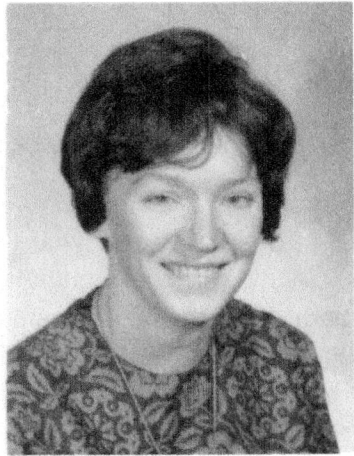

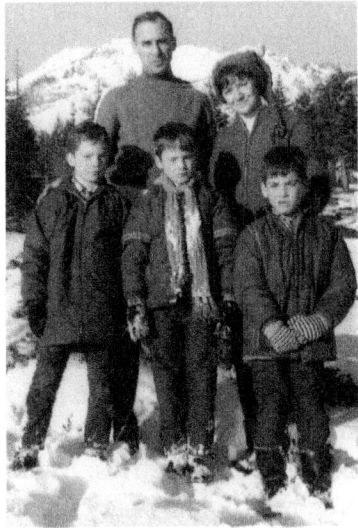

From left, Matt, Cal and Sabin(1966)

sense of how Gene wrote (and talked), here is what she wrote to them on the occasion of their 50th wedding anniversary, when they were both quite ill:

What we Geymans remember, overall, about you two, Pat and John, is the wonderful kindness that you have shown your friends and relatives. For us: in particular, we remember the generous "loan" of your cabin several times when our own vacation house was filled with full-time renters. The fun we had swinging on the heavy rope attached to the rafters (AT OUR AGE!) years ago. The time we took up your invitation to use your Mill Valley house one weekend—or maybe several times— but this time in particular, when we arrived at the empty house, alone, there was a tall, homemade chocolate cake awaiting, and a bottle of red wine! We remember our hikes together out toward Stinson Beach with such pleasure. Also, our heart-to-heart talks, friendly debates, at each others' houses, about life, kids, religion, politics (*@#%*). Values.......

We, still, try to emulate your: Strength Generosity Humor!

There is no one like either one of you for good, clear values, strong intelligence and, best: sympathy for the other guy. **Without getting mushy here**—*and skipping any number of adjectives and nouns that come to mind—I must report that neither John nor Gene have ever met two better people. Not before, not since. We send much love and admiration, on this, your 50th wedding anniversary.*

Gene had been raised in the Episcopal Church, and kept to tradition in marching our three boys off to the Episcopal church in Dunsmuir, just eight miles down the road to the south. Here is how they looked on such a journey one winter morning in the mid-1960s.

Gene was always game for a new adventure. Her enthusiasm, positive outlook, and buoyant nature were

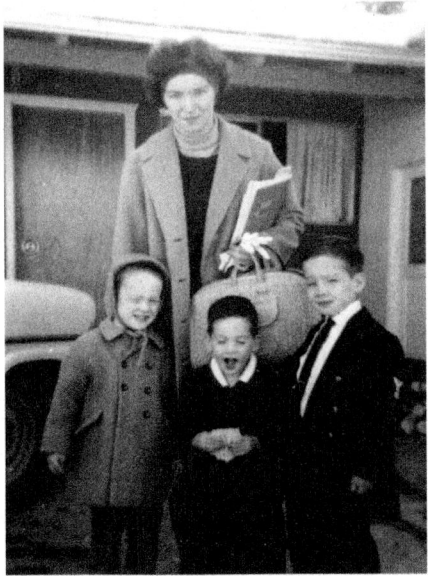

Gene and boys headed for church (from left, Cal, Sabin and Matt (1965)

just part of who she was. During our Mt. Shasta years I progressed in my flying, both airplanes and gliders, having run out of money during medical school after a $99 course to solo in the Bay area some years before. We had a club Cessna 182 at the local airport, and we made many trips to the Bay area and elsewhere—the whole family without a complaint. We made one trip to the Calaveras County Fair to enter our own frog (Shasta Sam) in the annual frog-jumping contest which continues since Mark Twain's early days there. It was a very hot day. Shasta Sam had to be resuscitated in a pond before his turn, then managed only four feet in three jumps!

The Mt. Shasta years were exciting and formative for the whole family. In later years, when our sons were contemplating marriage, this was always the place they would take their brides-to-be.

Why then did we leave? As a committed advocate for general practice as the foundation of our health care system, I had been involved in teaching medical students in my practice from the start. When family practice was recognized as the 20th specialty in American medicine in 1969, the next challenge was to build new education programs in U.S. medical schools and hospitals across the country. I could not resist the challenge, and soon found myself heading up the residency program where I had trained—Sonoma County Hospital—expanding it to a three-year program, and setting up an affiliation with UCSF medical school for both medical students and residents.

Once again, Gene took this move and later ones in stride, as she always had in earlier years growing up in her own family. What to do with her horse was a problem. For various reasons, I had gone ahead to Santa Rosa with our three boys a few days earlier. She ended up loading the horse in a trailer herself, then driving herself and horse all the way to Santa Rosa (more than 200 miles), arriving at night when a friend of ours—Scott Chilcott—showed us the way to a pasture several miles out of town. Typical Gene—what's the problem?!

Chapter 4

City Life and Full-Time Teaching

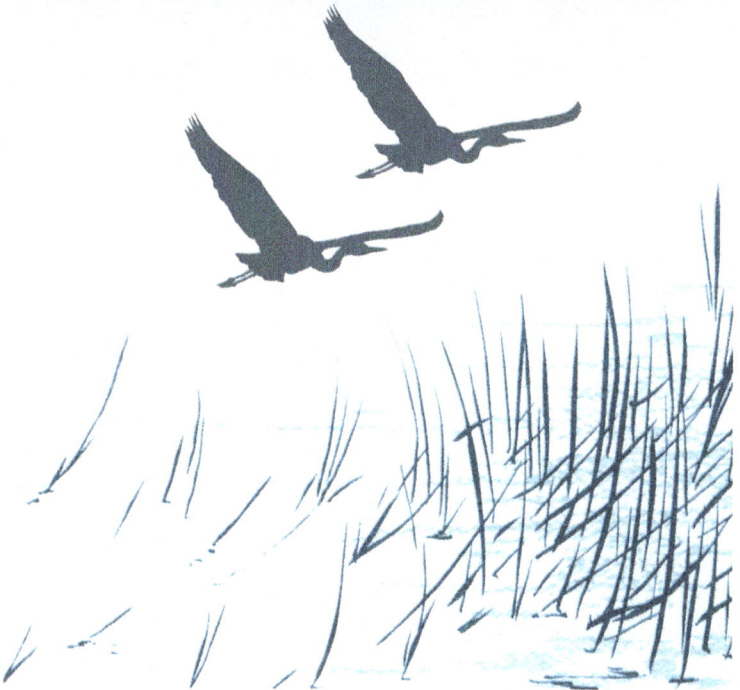

Our years from 1969 to 1990 involved a return to city life, which had been the norm for Gene throughout her life. I became fully involved in teaching at three different medical schools. Gene and I made about as many moves during those years as she had made growing up in her own family, but she thrived wherever she was, urban or rural.

Here I will spare you chronology of all of these moves, but will instead pick out three of her special things that portray her personality and spirit. Having been an English major and Art minor at U. C. Berkeley, she was always creative, artistic, an accomplished writer, and a dedicated reader. So here we will highlight some of her activities in puppetry, writing and reading.

Puppetry

Gene developed an early interest in puppets and story telling in childhood, read about them in different cultures, and blossomed into a gifted professional puppeteer from the early 1970s on. After working with a psychiatric social worker/puppeteer in Salt Lake City when we were at the University of Utah, she started her own group—The Geyman Puppeteers—soon after we moved back to the University of California at Davis. The group included all three of our sons as well as friends of Gene's for some shows. Cal and I built her stage, Cal did sound effects, while Matt and Cal played music for some shows.

Gene gave more than 200 puppetry shows in Davis in many settings, including schools, libraries, and churches.

She wrote her own stories, made all of her puppets, and gave workshops for budding puppeteers. She was knowledgable about the history of puppets around the world, and saw puppets as a way for spontaneous expression of feelings between people. In hand notes that I found recently in her papers I found these words about the values of puppets: *transmitters of culture; awaken sense of drama, artistry, history and language; of special value for shyer children; educational value for good health and right-minded behavior.*

In other notes:

> *If I could sum up what I wanted to impart to kids, it is—The world is full of things you might do or become. I don't care which of them you choose, I think you are wonderful and will support you in your choice. (A lot of parents in raising their kids say—Now, there is only one way, do it my way or you won't be much, or I won't like you.) One hopes to help children experience success early in life.*

In a Davis newspaper account of her puppetry, Gene had this to say:

> *Puppets are exaggerated and the stories are exaggerated. This is the art of puppetry. They show us our own feelings but in a lighter way that we can handle. The puppets express feelings the children might not be allowed to express themselves.*

And about the cultural value of puppetry:

> *I'm particularly interested in African stories. They have some wonderful myths that American children don't know very much about. It's like the Native American fables and the lovely Mexican stories. There are tons of them that haven't been done on canned TV.*

42

Gene used four different kinds of puppets, all of which she made herself—hand puppets, in which the hand is placed in a sock-like figure, rod puppets with rods attached to the figure, marionettes on strings, and shadow puppets. Our kids did the sound effects, as boys are fully prepared to do, such as clapping, shouting, coughing, laughing, thunder, running and dying!

Here are examples of stories for kids 9 and 10 years old:

The Three Billy Goats Gruff (a story in which a greedy wizard is out-witted by a dragon).

Ruthie and Lisa (the lament of a little sister, Ruthie, who is bossed around by her big sister, Lisa. Little sister finally solves her problems by getting a tiger!).

How to Trick a Wizard (a story about how Freddy, a poor boy, recovers his stolen gold from a mean old wizard with the help of a friendly dragon).

Joe the Bear and Sam the Mouse (about how these two unlikely animals become friends).

Here is one picture during our Davis years, Gene with Stella Starlight and Matt with the dragon.

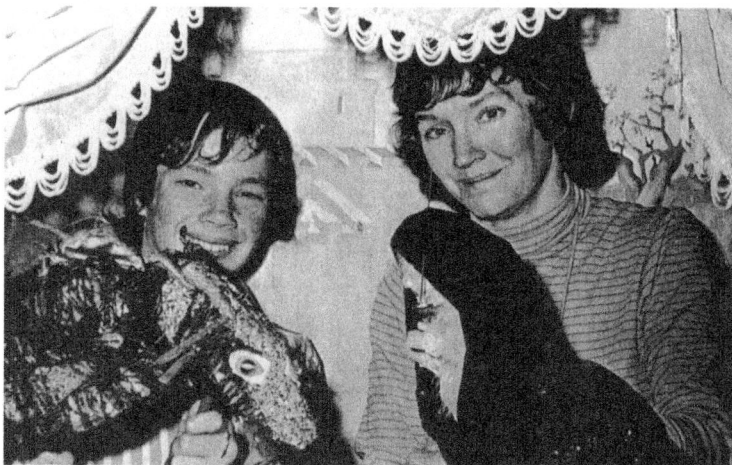

And they always had rapt audiences for their shows, as illustrated by this group.

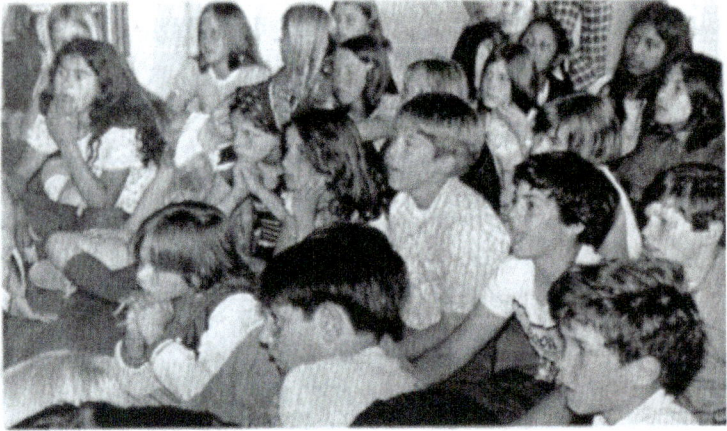

Gene gave puppet shows and workshops for puppeteers over some 30 years wherever we lived at the time, including after we moved to the San Juan Islands in 1990. After a show in the elementary school in Friday Harbor in 1992, her sack of puppets became lost, so she put out this announcement in Lost and Found:

2/15/92

LOST:

A sack of puppets –
a wizard in purple gown
a spider
a boy in a red cap
    – and others

– May have been lost at grammar school.   Call: 378-6264

Writing

Gene was a talented writer from high school on. She wrote for her high school paper in Marin County, California, where an English teacher, Katherine Martin, was an early mentor. Gene liked to do feature writing, and won a State of California award for creative writing. During the 1960s while we were in Mt. Shasta, she was a regular feature writer for the Mt. Shasta paper with many devoted readers.

She was also a poet, which I didn't even know until I discovered the following in a leather-bound diary she had kept in the first years after we were married. Imagine finding these words some 50 years later among her papers!

SOME PEOPLE

Isn't it strange
some people
make you feel so timid inside
your thoughts begin to shrivel up
like leaves all brown and dried.
But when you're with
Some other ones
it's strange still to find
your thoughts as thick as fireflies
all shiny in your mind.

ABOUT LOVE

Because of John Geyman
and other such people that I love . .
I love you
Not only for what you are
but for what I am when I am with you.
I love you
Not only for what you have made of yourself
but for what you are making of me.
I love you
For the part of me
that you bring out.
I love you
For putting your hand into my heaped up heart
and passing over all the foolish weak things
you cannot help knowing there
and for drawing out into the light
all the beautiful belongings
that no one else had looked quite far enough to
    find.

As I'm sure you will understand, these poems were a treasure for me to find some months after Gene died. I surrender to tears every time I read them.

Other excerpts of her writings over the years give us further insight into her thinking and spirit over the 56 years of our love story.

This from her diary in the spring of 1956 just before our marriage:

Now I am learning about love—it isn't physical at all but spiritual. Just a little bit, I can feel my soul touch John's. Our souls belong to God, and here on earth they can learn of God through perfect love of one another. . . . Such a delight in loving, as well as being loved! God is good to me. . . . Two things I must always hold in my heart all my life, if only six more minutes or sixty more years, is this: the essence of life is being—existing, and loving God. We live only half a life if we fear disease, war, accident and death—that is only for the timid. Living is exulting in life and love (which must be the closest expression that man can know of the Spirit of God) and accepting with gladness the unknown— Death. Thy will be done.

This from a 1980 article, published in a summer issue of *Family* magazine about puppetry, illustrates her charming and special writing style:

Sometime this summer—it happens every year—your children or grandchildren are going to collapse in the easy chair muttering, 'Oh man, what's there to do?'

Quick. Before they switch on the TV, bring on the puppets! . . . This much-loved folk art has other things going for it, besides keeping kids out of fist fights.

Growing brave backstage, shy children often become more self-confident in public. Impatient youngsters learn to slow down and e-nun-ci-ate. Educators view puppetry as a serious way to improve reading skills. And psychologists believe that puppets are a great release for scary feelings.

And, just to show how funny Gene has been throughout our lives together, this appeared on my bedroom dresser next to hers some 25 years ago:

Again: G.G. & J.G.!
I trust you notice that MY dresser is beautifully clean + well-ordered — whereas next to it, is this very dresser

During our years at the University of Washington, I flew gliders from the beautiful grass strip in Issaquah, just east of Seattle. Gene flew with me a number of times, closely watched the proceedings, and began incubating what became her excellent book, *Ghost Pilot,* a few years later. This back cover summary of the book by Jonathan Taylor, then president of the San Juan Pilots Association, describes what she accomplished:

[This book] completely engages the reader. The tale has all of the essential ingredients—interesting characters, trouble overcome, dramatic plot twists and a satisfactory conclusion. It is told against the dual and contrasting backdrops of a teenager's school and family life and the aviation environment in which he discovers his true potential.

Reading

From early childhood on, Gene always had a book in her hand. She was an inveterate reader, across all kinds of content, more fiction than non-fiction. She was a natural English major in college. Reading and writing were of one fabric.

As our joint library attests, Gene's reading interests were wide-ranging, including the classics, history, psychology, the natural world, and much more. We never discarded books, just accumulated more. We didn't miss many library book sales.

Here is one of her favorite poems that reflects her zest for life:[1]

When I Am An Old Woman I Shall Wear Purple

With a red hat which doesn't go, and doesn't suit me.
And I shall spend my pension on brandy and summer gloves
And satin sandals, and say we've no money for butter.
I shall sit down on the pavement when I'm tired
And gobble up samples in shops and press alarm bells
And run my stick along the public railings
And make up for the sobriety of my youth.
I shall go out in my slippers in the rain
And pick the flowers in other people's gardens
And learn to spit.

You can wear terrible shirts and grow more fat
And eat three pounds of sausages at a go
Or only bread and pickle for a week
And hoard pens and pencils and beer mats and things in boxes

But now we must have clothes that keep us dry
And pay our rent and not swear in the street

And set a good example for the children.
We must have friends to dinner and read the papers.

But maybe I ought to practice a little now?
So people who know me are not too shocked and sur-
prised
When suddenly I am old, and start to wear purple.

As is also my habit, Gene wrote all over her books. This is what she had to say about Ivan Doig's *This House of Sky: Landscapes of a Western Mind*:

Oh, I love his language. Wonderful verbs he uses. In a way, reading this book is like sitting down with a good friend and exchanging life stories.

In going through all of Gene's papers, letters, and writings in books, I naturally wanted to learn when her concerns about memory and Alzheimer's might have started. She did have an aunt who died of the disease. What I found is that her concerns started well before we finally dated its onset in about 1996. Though we had not talked about it at the time, among the many notes she made in a 1994 book, *50 Ways to a Better Memory* by Hermine Hilton, this section stands out:[2]

DEVELOP EAR-MINDEDNESS.

18

Even though the initial impact of seeing is said to be much stronger than that of any other sense, what we see is often not slated for longevity in the mind. The mind's ear is a much more important tool than the mind's eye. In fact, an auditory message to the mind's ear can bring about a visual image en route. For example, if someone tells you *not* to visualize a pink elephant, chances are you're already seeing one.

Even when names, numbers, and facts are seen printed on a card or written on a page, the letters and numbers don't really stimulate the mind's eye. But hearing those same names, numbers, and facts wakes up our memory machine. That is why the best approach to getting into the mnemonic habit is to become more ear-minded. Things register in our memory through our five senses. In most cases, seeing and hearing are the most predominant senses. People who feel they remember best what they see may think of themselves as eye-minded. People who remember best what they hear are ear-minded. A motor-minded person obtains memories through the remaining senses of touch, taste, and smell.

Yes, for sure (for me)

50

It turned out later that our son Cal recalled hearing Gene share her anxieties about possible future Alzheimer's well before the illness declared itself.

Chapter 5

Return to Rural Life:
San Juan Island

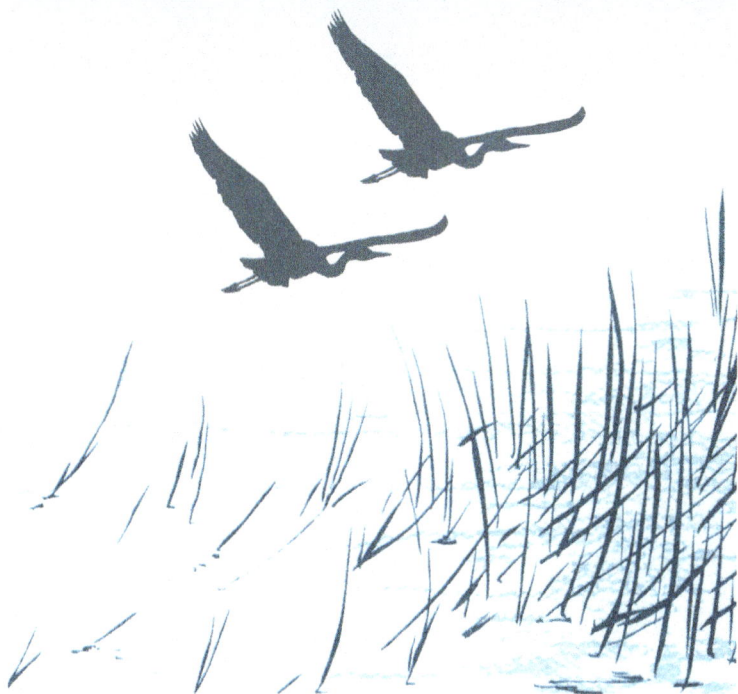

After almost **20 years** in cities, Gene and I were both missing the sense of community that we had come to enjoy in our Mt. Shasta years. We had lived in Salt Lake City, Utah, and Davis, California, followed by fourteen years in Seattle as I taught in universities and worked to develop family medicine programs in medical schools and teaching hospitals. Gene continued doing puppet shows and some teaching. When our son, Cal, graduated from Stanford University in 1981, we celebrated our 25th Aniversary by renewing our vows at the Stanford Chapel.

By the late 1980s, it was time to make some changes. Our kids had grown up, left home for college and moved on with their own lives, so downsizing made sense. We sold our house in Bellevue, just across Lake Washington from Seattle, and moved into a smaller condo a few miles north in Kirkland with a nice view across the lake.

Meanwhile we looked around the region for a small community where we could make a difference in our next chapter. We were especially interested in the San Juan Islands, looked at several of the islands, and soon decided on Friday Harbor on San Juan Island itself. With a population of about 2,500 in town and another 6,000 on the island, this was much like what we had known in Mt. Shasta. One important feature was the excellent airport there, including an instrument approach, since I did plan to fly back and forth to the University of Washington at regular intervals over the next few years.

We found a cabin on the west side of the island and

began flying there regularly on weekends. That gave us a chance to meet people, get involved in the community, and experience all four seasons before deciding where to live on the island. During that time we found that we were not condo people in Kirkland and began looking for a house large enough to accomodate family and friends during their trips to the island.

Our search soon focused on the west side of the island where we could see across to the Olympic Mountains, Victoria and Vancouver Island just across the U.S.-Canadian border. As Gene and I had so often done over the years, our decision on where to land was almost immediate and completely shared. The oak tree pictured on an opening page of this book, well over 200 years old with a common root for its two major parts, was just outside the front door of the house that we purchased. Without going in the front door, Gene walked down the hill to see what it all looked like. By the time she came into the house, her decision (and mine) was mostly made.

We moved to the Island full-time from Kirkland in 1990. As was our pattern, both of us soon became actively involved in community activities. Gene did some substitute teaching, puppeteering, working as an EMT, and helping with the County Fair. I practiced part-time at the Inter Island Medical Center, served on the Hospital District Board, and stayed involved with various part-time activities at the University.

Our house had been built in 1975 and had no downstairs bedroom. Since we hoped to spend the rest of our lives there, we soon decided to remodel the house, mainly putting in a downstairs bedroom and an expanded study for me. We figured that one upstairs bedroom would become Gene's study, while another could serve in future years as a place for a caregiver should that become necessary. You will later see that these best-laid plans could never come to fruition even after 21 years in the best house that we ever had. I would also later discover that a caregiver's room on the second floor is not a good idea when 24/7 caregiving help is required.

One humorous thing about this time was Gene's name change. Her mother, an Emogene, gave Gene the same name. But Gene never liked the name. So she waited until her mother died in 1992 to change it. That required a visit to the King County Courthouse in Seattle, where the judge questioned Gene for her reasons—what other aliases did she have? Was she running drugs? And so on. That made his day, and Gene became Eugenia, but still went by Gene.

We have both loved living on San Juan Island, and have found the community both nurturing and interesting—many talented people with varied backgrounds, some with continuity over generations and a strong sense of place, as extolled in Ivan Doig's writings.

As she did with everyplace that we had lived, Gene made our house special and personal as a reflection of both of our interests. Books all around, of course, beautiful use of color and space, though nothing very fancy. My mother had kept a large quilt in a cedar chest for many years after inheriting it from an aunt two generations earlier who had made it coming across the country in a wagon in 1847. That quilt ended up on a wall where we could live with it every day.

Our San Juan house was on a hill 330 feet above the water, facing south with a 180-degree view across the straits to the Olympics and Victoria. We had almost six acres to take care of, but most of it was natural with wildlife ranging from deer, foxes, raccoons and many birds to river otters that occasionally came up the hill from the ocean to clean out a neighbor's pond of fish. From our hilltop perch, we could see the storms coming across the

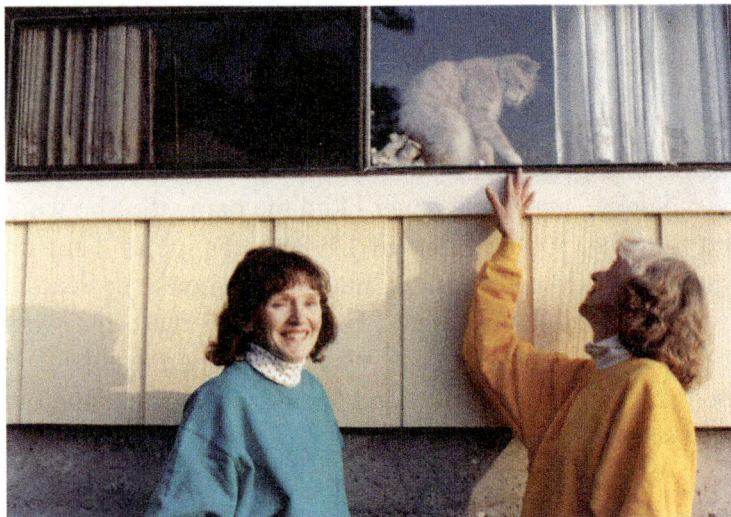

Gene and Carolyn with our cat Zeke at our San Juan house (1992)

straits. Fully exposed to frequent winds, we recorded gusts above 80 and 90 mph on occasion. With such winds, our window panes would move in and out so that Gene would use duct tape as Xs to protect them.

Since Gene had loved cats all her life from childhood on, a cat soon joined the family. Here Gene is with my sister Carolyn with one such cat in our early years on the Island.

This was also a great place for dogs, so Gent, a fine Chesapeake Retriever, also joined the family. As was her

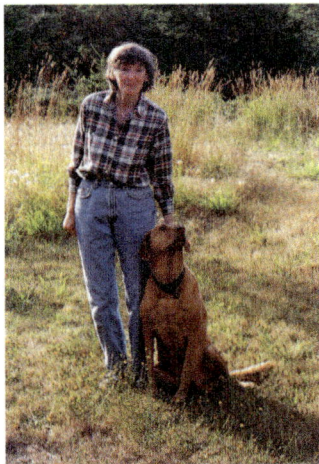

Gene with Gent, our Chesapeake Retriever (1995)

wont, Gene and Gent walked every day, and we took him swimming at island beaches on many occasions. Here they are just returning from a walk on our hill.

After Matt, our oldest son, married Amy Arvidson in September, 1991, at an old Island church dating back to the 1800s, the wedding reception was held at our house. Here is the family by the same oak tree that first attracted us to our hill.

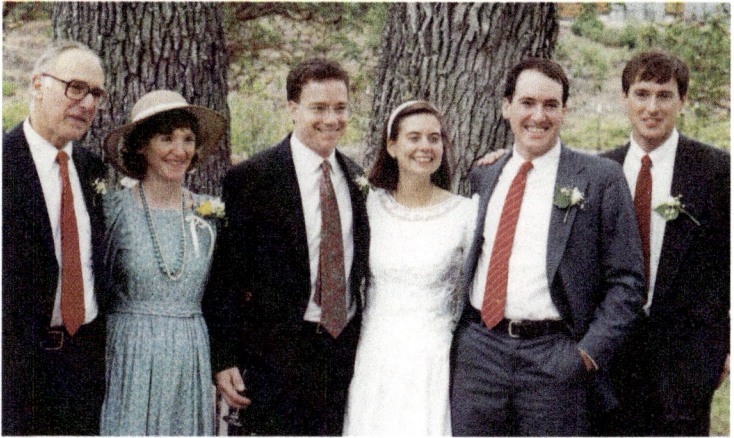

Wedding reception for Matt and Amy (from left, me, Gene, Matt, Amy, Sabin and Cal) (September 7, 1991)

Gene became fully occupied in many ways in our island community. She made friends easily, joined a regular hiking group and the Garden Club, and worked as an EMT. In that capacity, she participated in many emergency calls day and night, and soon distinguished herself as the one most willing to talk with other family members during a call. She was honored as EMT of the Year for her service in 1994. In those years she had no trouble finding call locations, even at night, on poorly marked dirt roads around the island. She also found time to volunteer at the San Juan Island Public Library. Here she is with one of her puppets at the Library (following page).

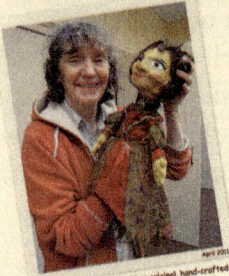

In the Spotlight

Meet San Juan Island Library Volunteer

Gene Geyman

She's an artist, puppeteer, and library book processor on Friday mornings!

April 2011

Gene Geyman is all smiles with one of her original, hand-crafted creations!

Gene with puppet at San Juan Island Public Library

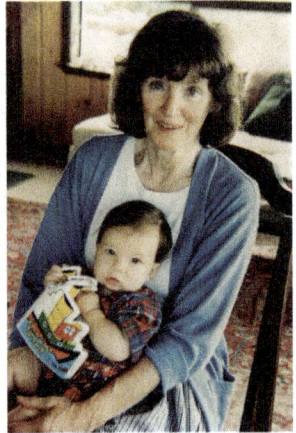

Gene with our first grandson, Ben (1996)

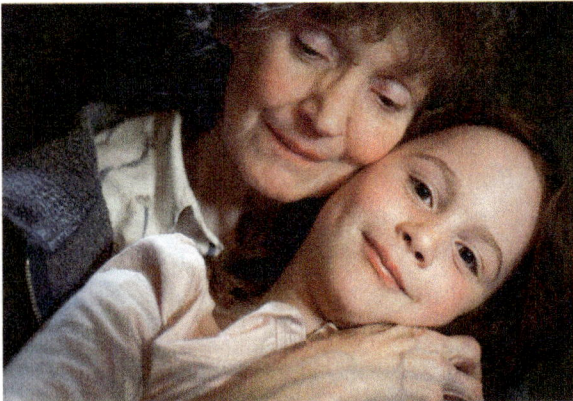

Gene with our fourth grand-child, Laura (2006)

As you'd expect, Gene was a loving and caring grandmother with Matt and Amy's children, Ben and Emily, and Cal and Lisa's children, Will and Laura.

Gene was also fond of calling herself their godmother. Most people wouldn't ask what that meant, but when one of our friends did, he got this response from Gene: "Whenever I say something, the kids just say 'Oh, God, mother!'."

Here's another example of Gene's ever-present surprising humor, from a 1994 letter to her favorite cousin Debbie at Halloween:

Up here, on the top of the tall hill where we live, the wind has been howling (up to 35 mph with gusts up to 45) non-stop for about twelve hours, and it does sound/feel like Halloween. I keep glancing out the window, hoping to catch sight of witches on broomsticks. So far, only see large black crows sailing past on ridge lift. I went to a friend's party last night as Raggedly Ann, wearing a home-made orange wig (from hunks of sheep wool), used lots of makeup; had made—poorly—a long-sleeved, flowered dress and a slightly shorter, long white apron.

Listen, I'm talking about a lot of work here. John, shy, would only wear a Frankenstein rubber mask from the local dime store, but STILL got the prize because no one guessed who he was (we didn't arrive together—seldom do, because of the medical call system up here on the island). (J. refers to it as "The Call." I refer to it as "The Clap.") Instead of saying a word at the party, he just lurched around making growly noises like a ten year old. Which took no work at all. And he won the prize. Alright, so the prize was just a pumpkin. I don't care . . . There is no justice.

The 1980s and 1990s were also times when we traveled quite a bit, much more than was possible after Alzheimer's became a problem. Most of our overseas trips were connected with my work in family medicine and rural healthcare, not as tourists. Gene was always interested in other cultures, their history and people, and was up for anything. During a five-week visit to Beer Sheva Medical School in Israel, we made a tour of the country to study their health care system. Here she is coming out of the water at Elat on the Red Sea after snorkeling. Ten years later, we were in Llasa, Tibet, on the occasion of the 30th anniversary of Tibet's only medical school, which confronts the ongoing challenge of training physicians and health professionals for a mostly rural country.

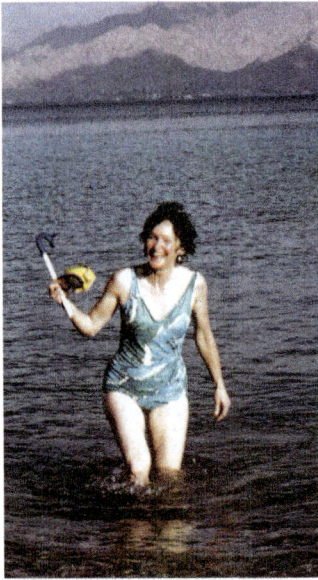

Gene at Elat on the Red Sea (1985)   Gene and I arriving at Llasa, Tibet (1986)

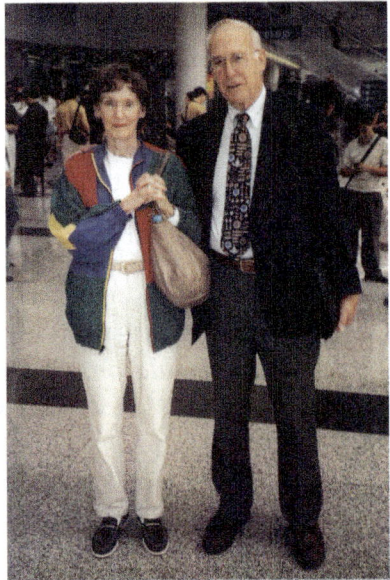

Much as Gene liked to travel, I soon learned that she was claustrophobic in commercial airplanes. That first became apparent in the 1960s, and later on I would give her a mild anti-anxiety drug to deal with it. This dated back to a bad experience in college at Berkeley when she was caught alone in an elevator between floors for four hours before a janitor realized the problem and got her out. She was never claustrophobic flying with me in small airplanes, but this became a lifelong problem whenever she felt she could not get out if she wanted to. As you will see later, this single event had everything to do with what kind of care she would accept with Alzheimer's. She was always too independent to tolerate being hemmed in by barriers she couldn't get around.

Much as I remained mostly unaware of Gene's worries about future Alzheimer's, she kept on doing all the "right" things to delay or prevent that problem—seeing people, remaining active, exercising, reading widely, and nurturing her garden. This poem (following page), protected by a laminated cover, lived on our bathroom counter for most of our lives together.

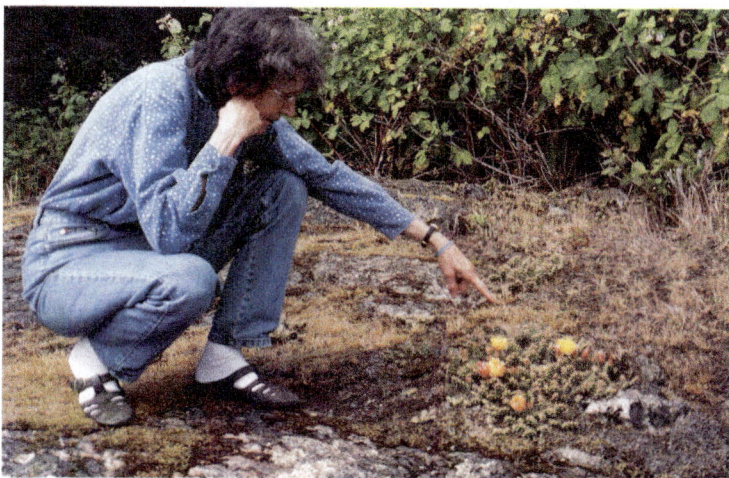

Gene pointing to a native cactus at our San Juan house

But despite all these efforts, Alzheimer's, the Great Thief, was just around the corner.

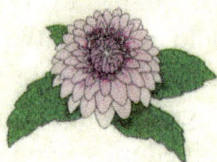

COLLECT

May the peace of my garden
Still my troubled hours,
May the beauty of my garden
Shine through my daily life.
May the dependability of my
garden
Teach me faith,
May the joyous colors of my
garden
Fill my heart with song, and
May my garden vision
Unfold the wings of my spirit.

PART II

Our Lives With Alzheimer's
(1996-2012)

Chapter 6

The Onset of Alzheimer's

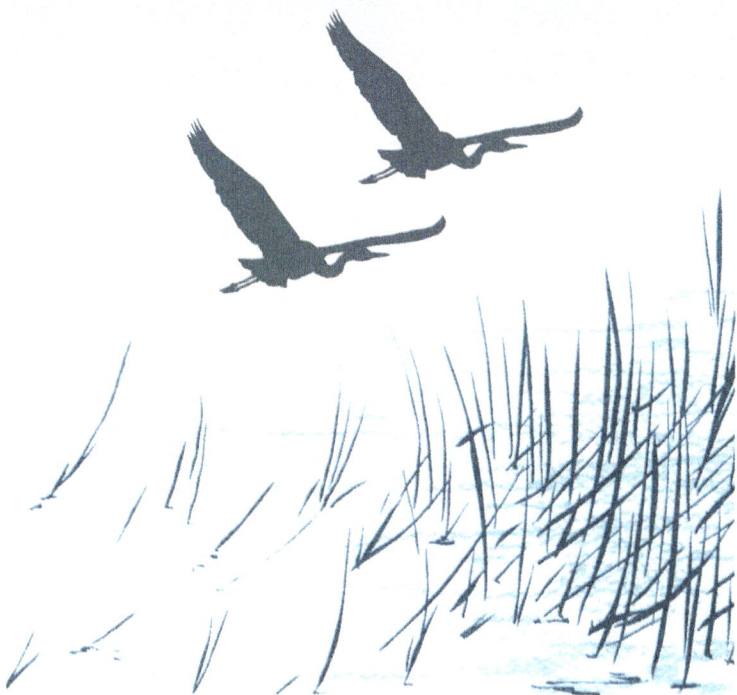

It all started so gradually as to be imperceptible at the time. As is true for most cases of Alzheimer's, it is easier in hindsight to date its actual onset. We all have lapses of short-term memory (join the club!).

The first sign of a new problem that I noticed goes back to 1996, when I was trying to teach Gene to fly our airplane. A logbook entry that year, that I had forgotten until recently, showed that we attempted several lessons to familiarize her with the controls and use of the radio. She had flown with me in various light airplanes for some thirty years. She had also taken a two-day pinch hitter course offered by the Aircraft Owners and Pilots Association in Seattle some 20 years earlier in an effort to gain enough skill to land the airplane in case I ever became incapacitated in the air. So she again wanted to upgrade those skills. As a certified flight instructor, I tried to get her used to the basic controls of the airplane. All to no avail—she just couldn't "get" what each of the controls do, and we had to abandon that effort.

A year later, my sister Carolyn noticed another early sign of Alzheimer's. She asked Gene to help with her move up to Seattle from a small coastal town in Oregon. Recall that they had roomed together in college, so they'd known each other well for many years. It took a couple of days for them to gather up her things for the trip back to Seattle. A key part of the move, of course, was to organize things into boxes and stacks that made sense for when she settled into her new place. Carolyn remembers that all her efforts to establish any kind of order would get shuffled around and changed by Gene, so they would have to keep doing it all over again. All just trying to help, but not quite understanding what it was about.

And the next year our son Matt noticed another kind of a cognitive problem during one of our visits to his home in Seattle. She had trouble undoing a latch on a garage door. This was the first time anyone had mentioned the name "Alzheimer's."

We are indebted to Dr. Barry Reisberg, professor of psychiatry at New York University School of Medicine, for his 1982 classification of Alzheimer's seven stages.

His *Stage 1* is without impairment. In *Stage 2*, people have memory lapses, such as forgetting familiar words and names or the location of keys, eyeglasses or everyday objects. But these lapses are generally not obvious to others or found during a medical examination.

Stage 3 has mild cognitive impairment (MCI), which is found in some 10 to 20 percent of people over 65 years of age. In fact, MCI to a certain extent is the norm in older people, with only one in a hundred avoiding it altogether over their entire lives.

At these early stages, changes are so subtle as to be easily overlooked. Then when they become more frequent, many of us tend to deny them.

While the course of individual patients with Alzheimer's varies widely, Dr. Reisberg tells us that MCI, on average, lasts about seven years before it interferes with activities of daily life.[1] As you will see farther along in our story, that estimate came quite close to Gene's situation.

As you have already read, Gene had been worried about possible future Alzheimer's for many years, probably because of an aunt's family history. But she also often said that she had been "absent-minded" as a child, with her mother often on her case about losing this or that.

In going back over the books that Gene was reading during these early years, she carefully read (and underlined) a number of books about memory. What she underlined was telling. In a 1999 book (which she had bought herself), *The Caregiver: A Life With Alzheimer's* by Aaron Alterra (a pseudonym),[2] Gene underlined a passage that with Alzheimer's, beyond loss of vocabulary is "the loss of the sense of how things are connected." In a 2001 book, *The Seven Sins of Memory: How the Mind Forgets and Remembers* by Daniel Schacter,[3] she identified with a passage dealing with not being able to remember names in order to introduce two people she knows well; she wrote this in the margin: "Yes."

Meanwhile she was doing everything possible to minimize the impact of what she by now knew was her early Alzheimer's (though she still was mostly not talking to me about it). She devoured Dr. Julian Whitaker's book, *The Memory Solution,*[4] with its 10-step program to optimize memory and brain function, especially noting useful approaches through diet, exercise and mental workouts. She read past sections on depression without note. In answering questions on a Social Readjustment Scale that evaluates stress levels, she gave herself a good score except for "some problem with memory." She also wrote a note to herself to "buy (and use!) yellow post-its."

Despite what was going on and what her inner worries may have been, she was almost always outwardly happy. Here she is in a typical pose in our kitchen, despite her labors with cooking (following page).

I first took Gene to a consulting neurologist in 1998. The complaints then were vague—occasional mild dizziness and some problems with memory. Her examination

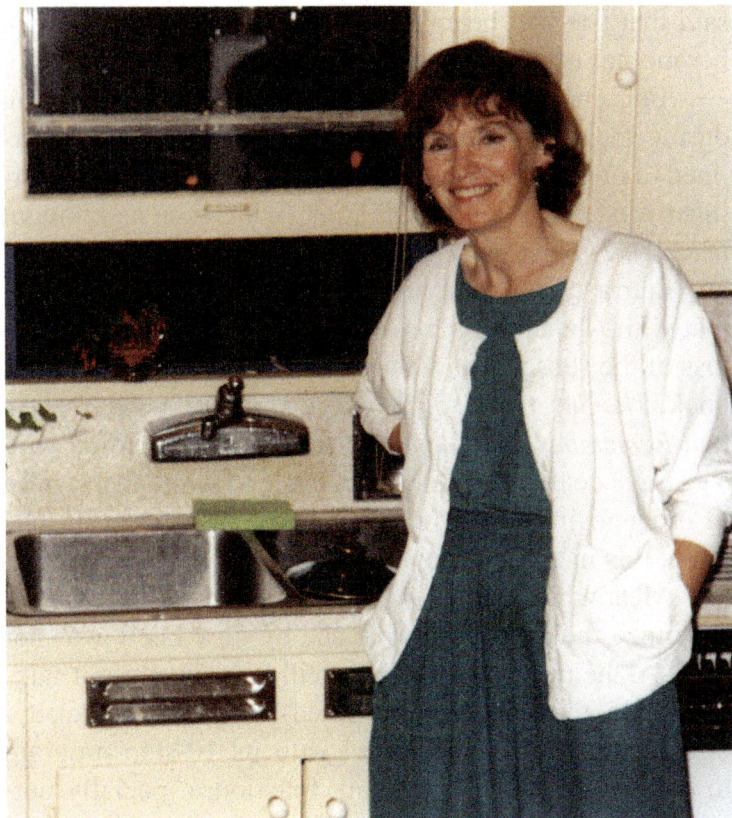
Gene in our kitchen

then was completely normal, as were her laboratory studies. She was still able to drive and to do all her activities of daily living. She remained active in the community, walked every day, and attended our local Fitness Center three days a week for aerobics. The only change we made was to add Tumeric, a supplement that may improve memory function, to her diet.

For the next three years, Gene's course was fairly stable. Most people would not notice cognitive and memory problems that were progressing very slowly.

So that's how it all started.

Chapter 7

Initial Treatment and Care Plan

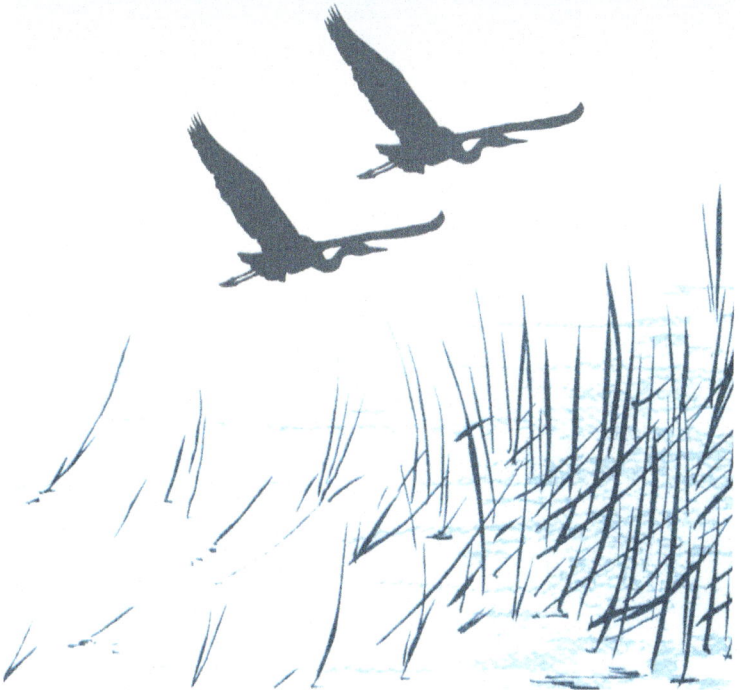

By now I could see the writing on the wall. I needed to develop a new life plan around the care of Gene's Alzheimer's that would work best for both of us.

The first basic question, of course, was where we should live as her disease predictably advanced. My hope was that we would be able to stay in our house on the west side of San Juan Island—that we both loved—where we could look out across the water to Canada and the Olympics and see the sunsets until we both went west ourselves. That had been our hope from the beginning, planning as we had for an upstairs caregiver bedroom and adding our own bedroom downstairs so we could stay on the ground floor when we could no longer manage stairs. At first I also thought that it wouldn't be too much of a problem to bring in caregivers there when I needed more help. (We will see later that the best laid plans . . . !)

It was also time to get a better handle on just where her disease had taken her already. Still mostly happy and engaged in the community, she was able to cover most of her problems with people not noticing much. At our ages, we're all in the same, growing club with senior moments!

Further examination and testing by her neurologist was mostly unremarkable, though her mini-mental status scores were starting to slip. The MRI added no new information, and she hated the noise and confinement of the procedure. She was referred for psychometric testing and spent several hours with a Ph.D. specialist in that area. His report was true but tactless and brutal for her to hear—"Don't write another book, do no more writing." It was hard for both of us to sit through his detailed explanation of how poorly she had done on all of the psychometric tests.

By now there was enough memory and cognitive change to warrant ongoing medication, so Gene started taking Aricept with the hope that it might at least delay the progression of her disease. She tolerated it well, but often questioned whether follow-up visits to the neurologist were needed. After one such visit a couple of years later, she didn't want to go back, saying she didn't like him and that "he looked at me funny."

Meanwhile, of course, we were pursuing other important parts of her care, including a regular exercise program at the Fitness Center, daily walks with the dog, seeing friends regularly, and staying as active as possible in the community.

I knew that her future course would be partly unpredictable, but also progressively downhill. We would try to enjoy each stage as much as possible. My roles as husband, caregiver and physician (now retired from practice) cut several ways. I resisted keeping a diary of progression as "too clinical" (and did not do so until the last year and a half of her life, when more rapid changes required an accurate overview to pass on to her treating physicians).

In those early years of her disease, I tried to look ahead at nodal points that we would likely confront down the track, wondering at what point I might need to transfer her care to full-time shift caregivers, perhaps even in a long-term care facility. These are the nodal points that occurred to me at that time as potential future gamechangers:

- When Gene could no longer drive.
- When I had to make all the decisions, including her business affairs.
- When she could no longer use the telephone.
- When it was unsafe for her to be alone.
- If she wandered and got lost.
- If she became paranoid about people or groups.
- If violent or combative behavior became an unresolvable problem.
- When she couldn't manage activities of daily living at home.
- When we would need 24-7 caregiver shift care.
- When she no longer knows who I am.

Beyond those junctures, of course, I was also aware of studies that have documented the increasing prevalence of depression among caregivers, together with shortening of their lives by several years. Since Gene would be worse off if I became incapacitated or died before her, this also became part of the equation.

Looking back on all of this, I made another big change (though I actually didn't realize it at the time) that in retrospect made it much easier for me to take on an increasing role as caregiver. In 1997, (soon after we later documented the onset of Gene's Alzheimer's), Gene took a five-week trip to Switzerland and France with a couple we had known well during our Mt. Shasta years. I had plenty of time looking out to Canada and the Olympics during those five weeks to ponder our future. I had practiced family medicine on San Juan Island since 1990, but made a big decision about my own life during that time. Much as I had enjoyed practice, I decided to shift gears and enter my own next chapter of research and writing on the health care system, a subject that had interested me for many years. I could not do that and still maintain an active practice, so I decided to make the change.

It soon became apparent that was the only way I could do my work and be Gene's caregiver at the same time. From my study at home, I could do almost all of my work, be aware of what was happening with Gene, and be there if any problems arose. She kept active in gardening, was still cooking and able to drive. Here she is on an especially happy day with her new Chevy in 2001.

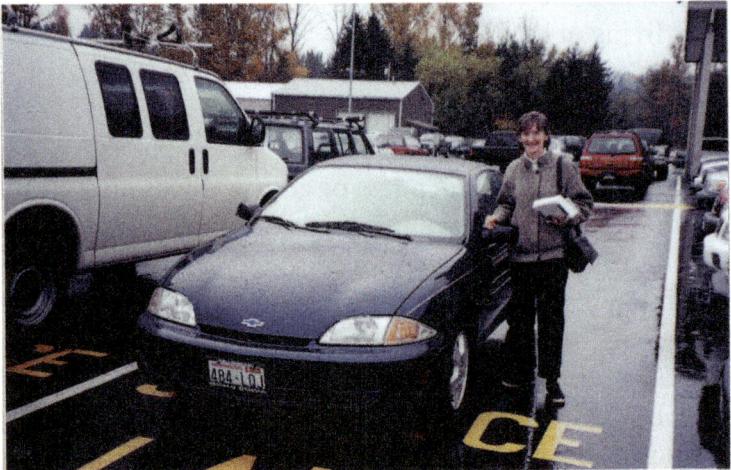

Gene's new car (2001)

As we moved toward new challenges ahead, Gene and I treasured her independence. Both of us knew that it wouldn't last but were still not using the word Alzheimer's in our everyday conversation. But the Great Thief was ever present, as we will soon see.

CHAPTER 8

Subtle and Relentless Progression of Alzheimer's

Life is what happens when you're not looking.
—John Lennon

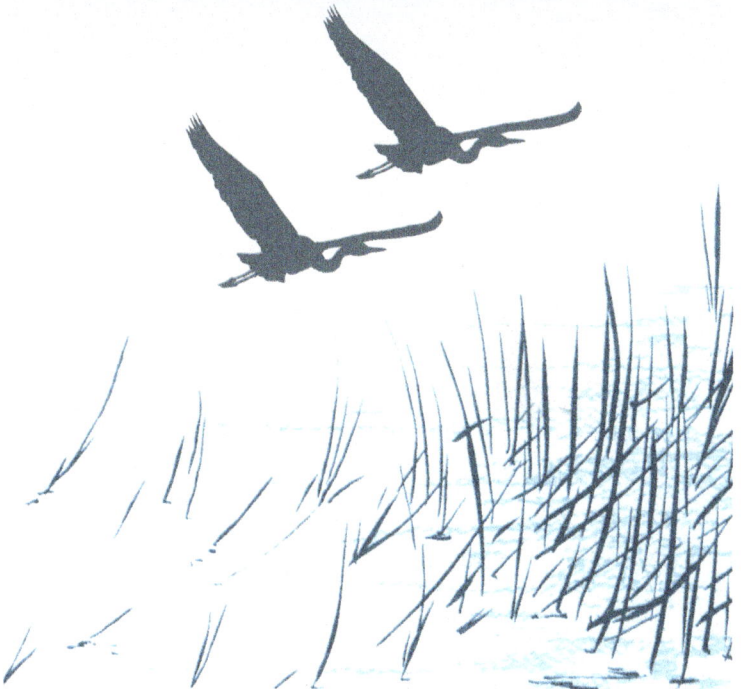

As we all know, Alzheimer's advances in unpredictable ways, different for every patient, but relentless just the same. For Gene, the period from 2001 to 2009 was marked by periods of relative stability punctuated by episodes of declining function. Overall, during those eight years, she progressed from Stage 3 to Stage 5 as categorized by the Alzheimer's Association.

These are the highlights of these three stages:

Stage 3:

Friends, family or co-workers begin to notice deficiencies. Problems with memory or concentration may be measurable in clinical testing or discernible during a detailed medical interview. Common difficulties include word- or name-finding problems noticeable to family or close associates . . . reading a passage and retaining little material . . . losing or misplacing a valuable object . . . decline in ability to plan or organize.

Stage 4:

A careful medical interview detects clear-cut deficiencies . . . decreased knowledge of recent occasions or current events; impaired ability to perform challenging mental arithmetic— for example, to count backward from 75 by 7s;

*decreased capacity to perform complex tasks, such
as planning dinner for guests, paying bills and
managing finances; reduced memory of personal
history; the affected individual may seem subdued
and withdrawn, especially in socially or mentally
challenging situations.*

Stage 5:

*Major gaps in memory and deficits in
cognitive function emerge. Some assistance with
day-to-day activities becomes essential. At this
stage, individuals may be unable during a medical
interview to recall such important details as their
current address, their telephone number or the
name of the college or high school from which they
graduated . . . become confused about where they
are or about the date, day of the week or season.*

Each downward episode in Gene's course was usually subtle at the time and tended to blend in over months
to the point it was difficult to pin down until quite a bit
later. But what became obvious is that over a longer period they became a fixed pattern until other kinds of decline came along.

These are some of the markers of Gene's advancing
Alzheimer's between 2001, when she started medication
in earnest, and 2009.

- *She kept losing things, especially her purse and
  her glasses.* This started more on a daily basis, but
  later became many times each day. I purchased a
  Key Ringer (on Google), which gave us a way to
  find her purse almost all of the time. I kept trying
  to get her to wear her glasses around her neck, but
  that never came to pass!

- *She increasingly would repeat things she had said just a little while before.*
- *She had increasing difficulty with schedules,* to the point that I had to schedule everything.
- *Using the telephone became more difficult.* After a while she could not take messages and would often have trouble dialing numbers.
- *She had problems with directions while driving.* I recall a time when I was driving to town and saw her driving in the other direction on a road that she seldom took. I turned around and followed her for miles. When she finally stopped, she had no idea where she was. This was painful to see since she had driven all of our island roads, often at night, in previous years as an EMT and never had had this kind of trouble.
- *Declining scores on the Mini-Mental Status exam* during office visits to her physician.

There were other general areas of concern over this eight-year period. Though she had always had an easy outgoing personality, she started to withdraw from groups and to talk less around people. Conversation became more difficult. Her favorite time during the week was working as a volunteer at the San Juan Island Public Library. She always enjoyed that and seeing colleagues on a regular basis, but talked less and started to have problems with some of the techniques used in processing books.

At home she would use her study less and less. She had her own computer, which she used a bit in the earlier years to write. But that became impossible, and she never could get on to email.

It was hard to watch Gene's continued decline, which of course frustrated her immensely. These are some of the more poignant moments.

- During one of her Mini-Mental Status tests, she thought long and hard how to answer the question "Where are you now?"; she finally answered Mt. Shasta, not Friday Harbor, where she had lived for more than 15 years.
- She started confusing, repetitively, cat food with bird food. Neither the cat nor the birds ever figured it out either!
- Since she was always worried about losing her purse at the Fitness Center during water aerobics, we tried to get her a locker and way to lock it up when she was in the pool; but she could never get the concept of using the key to open her locker.
- As a former English major and inveterate reader, I started to notice that she usually wasn't actually reading much, even with a book in front of her.

Another big change in our lives involved travel. We had traveled widely throughout our marriage, sometimes in groups such as the Citizen Ambassador Program to such places as China, Russia and Scandinavia, at other times to Israel and Tibet. But as her illness progressed, travel became much more of a problem. She would not want to fly in a commercial airliner. She would still fly with me, but the logistics of travel became too confusing. Our last trip down to the Bay Area in California was very confusing for her. Even while staying with family or friends of forty-plus years, she would not know where she was and wanted to go home—*now*!

In later years, maybe eleven or twelve years into her Alzheimer's (times blend, and it's hard to recall), Gene would point to her head and ask me "What's wrong up here?" At first my response was that she had some memory problems. Later I would call it Alzheimer's by name, and describe that a bit. But we would always end up saying that we all have our problems (she had helped me through my cancer in 1982 and heart attack in 2001), and that we would get through this together.

Many things became problems during these years, some of which were humorous. One of these was shopping. We would go to the grocery store together, each with our own list of what to get. When we met at the checkout stand, she would have the things on my list and a few other things. On some occasions, I could "lose" her in the market—I could look everywhere and not find her if she was behind an aisle as I kept looking!

Despite all these examples of a downward course of her Alzheimer's, life went on and we had many happy times. She especially enjoyed her work at the Library, including giving some puppetry performances for children. She worked in our garden as she could, and walked with friends and our dog, We would always have a glass of wine in the evening, listen to music and often danced. We had our 50th anniversary in 2006, nine years into her illness, and this was a very happy occasion. The collage of pictures (page 88) traces each of our lives from about age four to before and after our marriage.

As her illness progressed, I kept wondering how much insight Gene had. I found that difficult to figure, and was probably underestimating it. One example of that was her bringing up the subject of what I would do if she died first. I always dismissed that possibility since I was four years older and had already "died" once with my cardiac arrest and heart attack on my 70th birthday while she was in otherwise generally good health. She kept bringing the subject up, each time urging me to remarry if she died first. We would usually end that conversation by agreeing that we wanted to go at the same time.

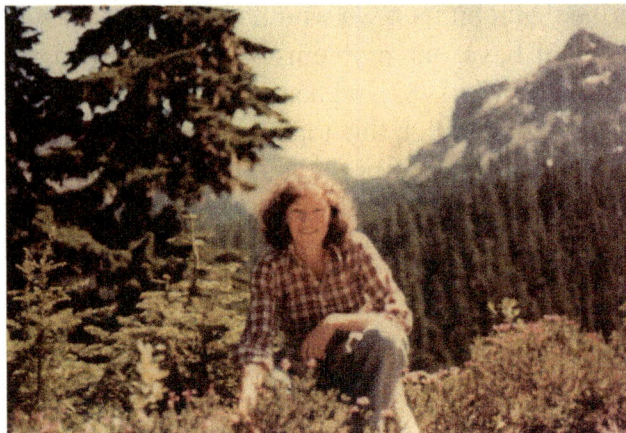

Gene on a hike
in the Cascades
(1990)

Her favorite place on
our deck, of course
with a book

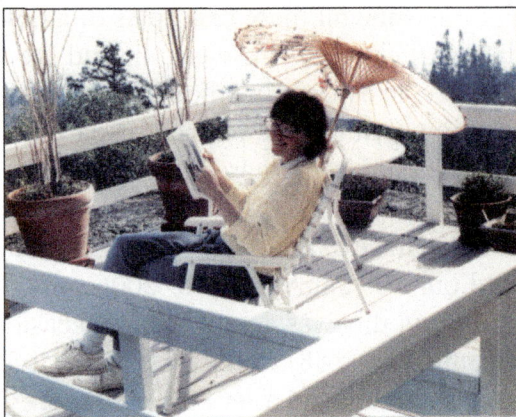

Gene, always a
gardener, bringing
plants to life

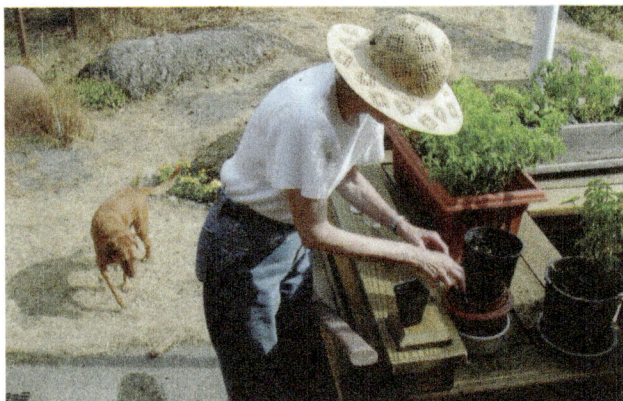

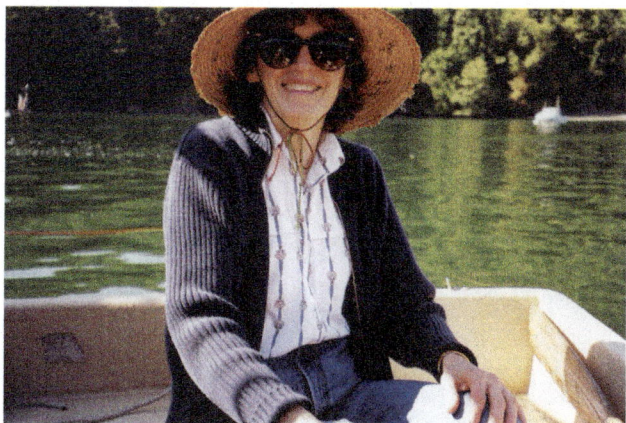

Gene on the water

Gene's note about Alzheimer's
(about 2001)

"Trouble City: My memory is not so hot nowadays. Have to write notes to myself as to what I'm going to/should do today, etc. Hope it doesn't get any worse. Going to go to a specialist in 8 days, see what's up."

Her beautiful smile always,
despite Alzheimer's

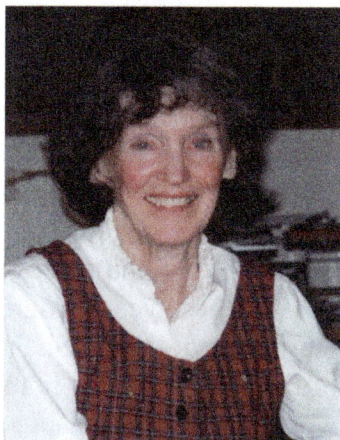

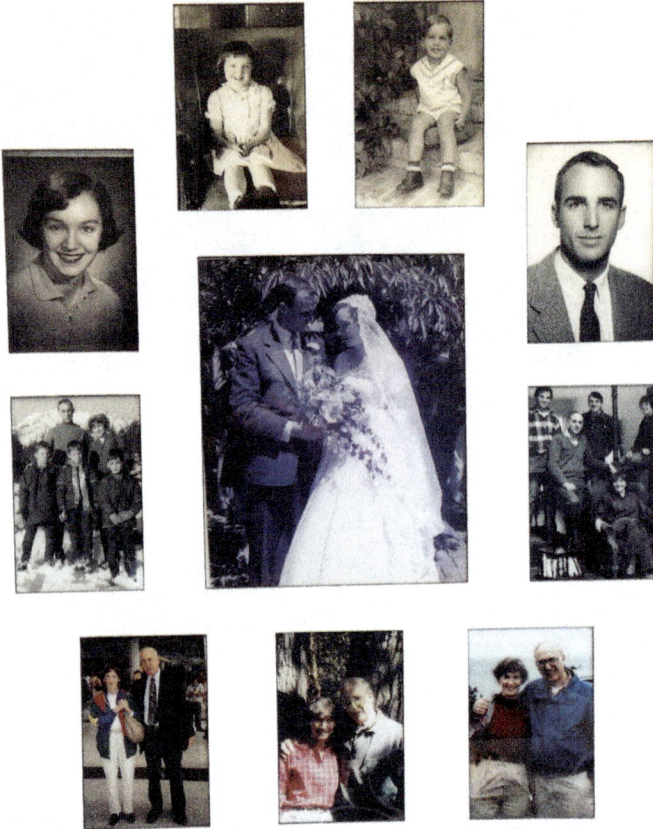

With each slide in function, Gene naturally became more dependent on me. We had always had a very close marriage, and we became ever closer. The more things she couldn't do, the harder she tried and the more I loved her. My goal was to support her all the way, be there for her, and *never* show disappointment.

As these years progressed, Gene started to get more fearful about things. She started to tell me she was afraid of being alone in the house and concerned that someone would break into the house. We changed our locks at least three times, and I started to wonder how long we could stay in the house we loved so much, nine miles from town. She was still driving, but that was soon to change.

Chapter 9

Losing Her Car

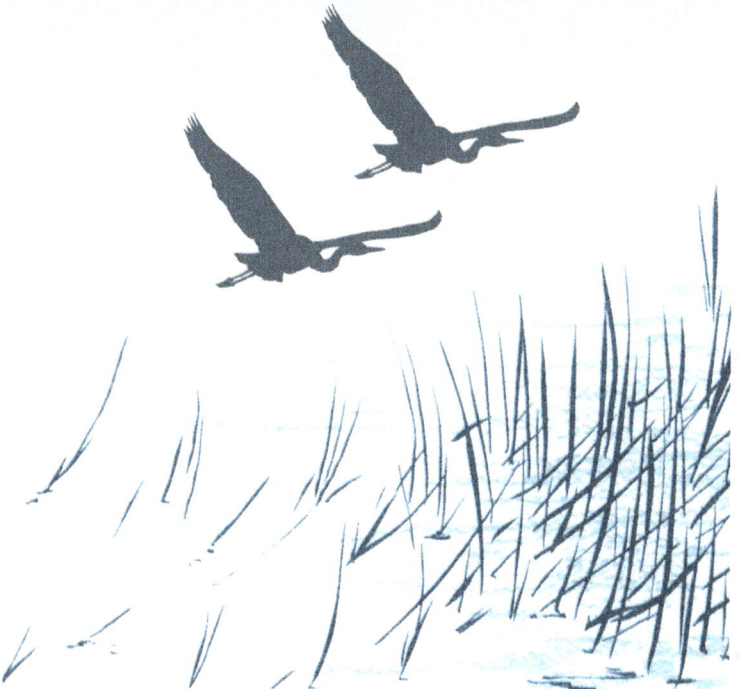

By 2009, in the thirteenth year of Gene's illness, she had lost her purse many hundreds of times, now on a daily basis. But one day the *Key Ringer* could not locate it. A long search everywhere revealed no purse. The trouble was, of course, that with the purse went her driver's license.

So we scheduled a time to renew her driver's license at the local DMV office. She had to retake the written exam, so we started reading the manual that updates all the procedures and regulations. She would need to achieve a 70 percent score to pass the test.

After studying for many days, including my quizzing her along the way, she could only manage 30 percent on the test. We went back after more study over another couple of weeks only to score 30 percent as before.

So there went the driver's license. She wanted to keep driving without a license. I didn't want to take that risk, and knew that by this time she had a lot more trouble with directions. So, though not entirely a joint decision, we marched down to the Island car dealer and sold her car the next day.

She was angry with me over that for quite a long while. As we all know, driving one's car is the last vestige of our own independence, so this was a big—but necessary loss. We now had just one car in the family, and we lived nine miles out of town, the central place on our Island.

My schedule was flexible and I worked from home, so we just planned to fully coordinate our schedules. My goal was to facilitate all of the things she liked and wanted to do. We would drive to town most days, and I just adapted to her times in town by working in my small hangar office at the airport. That worked out just fine.

Gene's anger about the car gradually resolved as she came to understand that she should no longer drive. As the months went on, she would often wonder where we were and say how amazed she was that I knew the Island roads so well. Recall that just a few years earlier she had driven all these roads alone as an EMT, plus other smaller dirt roads all over the Island, even at night.

In the aftermath of losing her car and much of her own independence, I was on the alert for signs of depression. These were not long in coming, so we soon started her on a small dose of an anti-depressant while endeavoring to maintain as much contact with people and community affairs as possible. But as expected, this was just the start of more problems ahead.

Chapter 10

Anxieties and Delusions

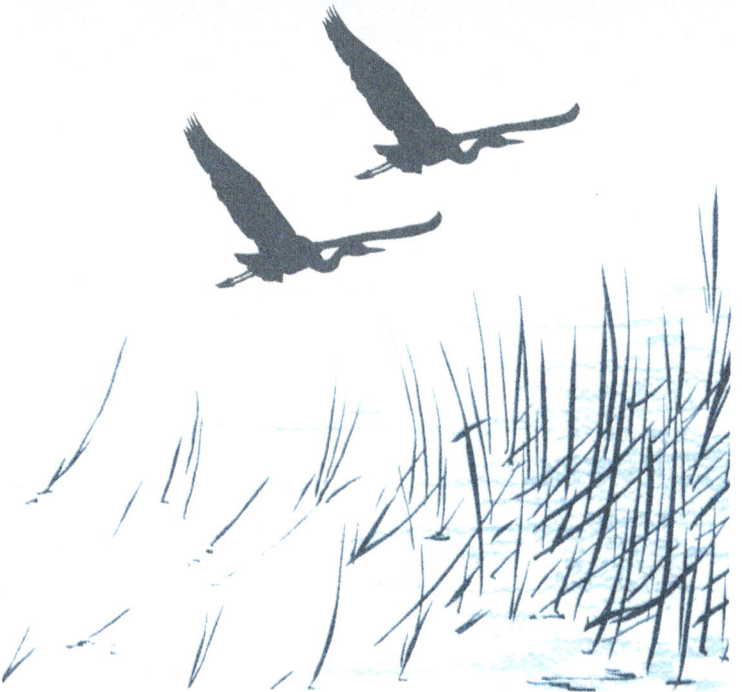

After Gene lost her car, everyday life became more of a struggle for us both. She was increasingly beset by new fears, anxieties and even delusions. We were entering the Alzheimer's Association's *Stage 6*:

Memory difficulties . . . worsen, significant personality changes may emerge and affected individuals need extensive help with customary daily activities. At this stage, individuals may lose most awareness of recent experiences and events as well as of their surroundings. . . occasionally forget the name of their spouse or primary caregiver but generally can distinguish familiar from unfamiliar faces . . . need help getting dressed properly; without supervision, may make such errors as putting pajamas over daytime clothes or shoes on wrong feet . . . have increasing episodes of urinary or fecal incontinence. . . experience significant personality changes and behavioral symptoms, including suspiciousness and delusions (for example, believing that their caregiver is an impostor); hallucinations (seeing or hearing things that are not really there); or compulsive, repetitive behaviors such as hand-wringing or tissue shredding.

In coming months, Gene was to experience most of these problems. The one I especially feared was incontinence, for I knew that that would require more care than I would be able to provide and perhaps leaving our home of 20 years that we so loved.

Gene was having increasing problems with conversation, finding words and completing sentences. Despite my knowing her so well, it became harder to decipher what she was trying to say. She was also losing confidence in conversation, and was starting to withdraw from groups of friends. When others in a group would dominate the conversation, she would become quietly angry and leave early if she could.

There were other behavioral changes as well. She became confused about dates and time, and could no longer plan a day. She could not use the TV remote and had difficulty tracking movies or TV. She was starting to read less, even though she often had a book in her hands. I would pass along the latest issue of *The New Yorker* (one of her favorites for years) and a daily newspaper, but these would go unread. And when we went to the Medical Center for her appointments, I would have to sign her name.

But she kept trying, doing what she could every day. She could still cook, do things in the garden, and always make our bed in the morning. Meanwhile, though, there were increasingly disorganized piles of clothes on the floor in our bedroom and cat/dog hairs and dust were accumulating all over the house!

She was becoming more fearful, even paranoid of some things. She was worried that some of our neighbors or others were breaking in and stealing her purse (by now it went missing virtually every day until the *Key Ringer* found it). She would tell me that various neighbors had moved or died. She awoke one night with a dream that we were the only two people on our entire Island (which is

20 by 10 miles with more than 6,000 people), and wanted to get off our "rock" right away. For the first time, she didn't know who I was. While in one of our nightly cuddles in bed, she asked "Who are you. Where are you from?", then became sullen.

With all this going on, she became further withdrawn and more depressed. After a long talk (and listening on my part attempting to figure out where she was), I heard suicidal ideation for the first time—"I'm stuck here, in this house, no friends, no car, my life is over."

That triggered an immediate response. We increased her anti-depressant and added Zyprexa, an anti-psychotic, in a low dosage avoiding any toxic side effects but still controlling her delusions. I went through the house and took all knives elsewhere for safe-keeping. I also decided to see if Gene would accept another caregiver in the house.

One woman had taken care of our dog for more than ten years, especially when we were traveling off-island. Gene knew her well and always liked her. So we asked her to come as a test when I visited my sister overnight in Seattle. At the start, Gene didn't recognize her until she smiled, but then they had a good time in their "slumber party" and hugged when she left the next day.

My next test of an overnight caregiver did not go so well, though I thought it was well planned. Again I tried to be off-Island for a day while Gene's brother Mike and sister-in-law Anne were here. Anne would stay in our house with Gene overnight. Her visit started out fine, but after a while Gene became strongly insistent, even combative, that Anne should leave— "I can manage in my own house... I've stayed here lots by myself... Why do I need help? Go home to your own house... When's John coming back?"

Despite all this turmoil, Gene kept her strong sense of self, as illustrated by this picture in our kitchen. She had often struck this pose, usually in jest, but now it was serious. And as events were changing more rapidly, I finally overcame my reluctance to keep a journal, which became a necessity.

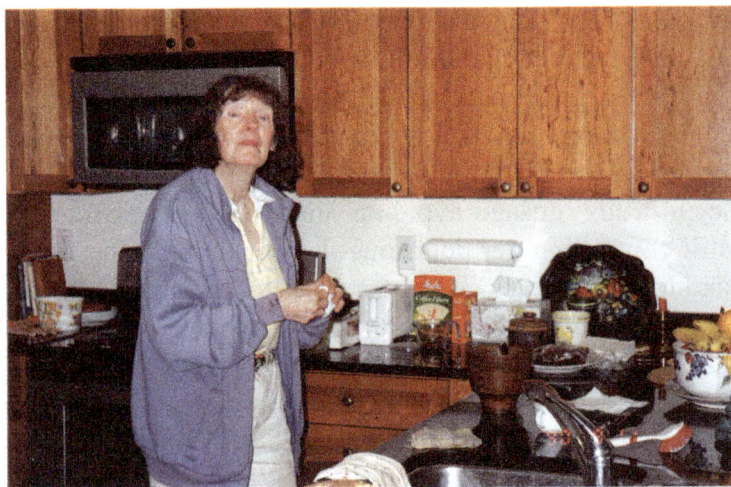

Determined to deal with her disease

Chapter 11

The Near-House Fire

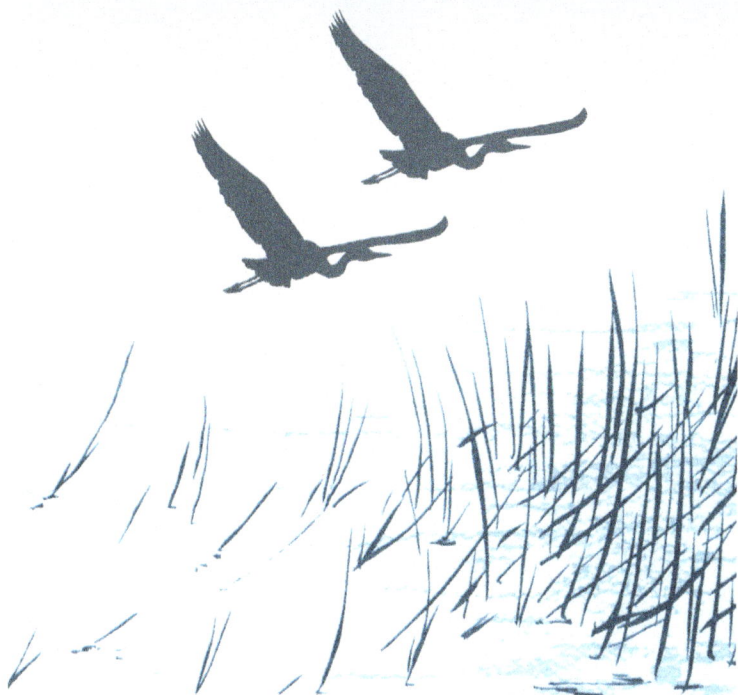

It happened late one afternoon just before Thanksgiving in 2010. I was in my study, on the ground floor of our San Juan house one room and about 30 feet from the kitchen where Gene was starting dinner for us. I came around the corner into the kitchen to find a solid wall of billowing smoke filling the room and moving into the next room. Gene had left something in the microwave, which was getting close to igniting, and she had no idea what to do. Her face was blank as she just looked at the smoke. She had no idea how to pull the plug, no longer knew about 911, and could not have called out anyway. A fire extinguisher was in an adjoining closet, but there was no way that she could have operated that.

This really got my attention. After getting everything turned off and clearing the house of smoke, it was time to rethink our whole plan of staying in the house nine miles from town. I first resolved that I should take over the micro-waving, and promptly installed a child lock on it. I also planned to watch more closely what was happening with the stove, thinking that Gene's days of cooking were probably numbered.

But the bigger question was what to do next? Should we move to town? Should we get more help in this house? Should we consider moving off Island to some kind of a progressive care place?

The last question was the easiest to answer. We had lived on San Juan Island for the last 21 years, the longest either of us had been anywhere in our lives. We had many friends in this nurturing community. And we had seen over the years many friends leave, usually because of health problems or to move closer to their children, where things did not work out as well as expected. The common underestimated factor seemed to be the loss of their support system and sense of community that they had enjoyed on the Island.

So we both agreed to stay on the Island. But to stay here in this house seemed impossible. Our nearly six acres were harder to maintain, and we certainly didn't need 3,200 square feet of house. It would be hard to get enough help here to spell me when I was in town. Our neighbors were not as close by as would be the case in town. The eighteen-mile roundtrip drive to and from town was getting fatiguing for me, especially if several times a day. And I could no longer in good conscience leave Gene alone in the house.

The writing was on the wall—find a smaller place in town, preferably within half a mile of downtown so that Gene could walk there, with an upstairs bedroom for a caregiver. As part of that same decision, I had to consider whether that would be a longer-term solution as well. What if the next step were to be incontinence, combative behavior or some other reason requiring around the clock nursing care? Again town had some answers—an assisted living facility with small space for an individual or couple and a nursing home (that included a locked Alzheimer's ward), but neither of us was ready to consider these possibilities.

While we were moving into this next phase of our lives, we tried to enjoy the last weeks in our house. This was an especially confusing and disorienting time for Gene. We were now using a higher dose of the Zyprexa to control her intermittent angers, disorientation and delusions. Life had become not just hour to hour but moment to moment. I tried never to leave her alone and watched the kitchen more closely (as a non-cook myself!). And we often listened to music and danced in the evenings.

Little more than a month after our near-house fire, Gene didn't know it was Christmas. I gave her a red robe, her favorite color, but a few hours later, she couldn't remember that and thought it had been in the closet for 25 years.

Though the need to move to town was obvious, Gene naturally had mixed feelings about it. We would both miss our house, the view, and the land we knew so well. But Gene was more fearful of being alone, and would welcome closer neighbors. At the same time, the whole idea of such a move was too much for her to understand, and it was clear that I would have to do all of the planning and arrangements for the move.

The next three months were more than busy. We looked at six possible places in town. One seemed to meet our needs quite well—a 1,600 square-foot two-story townhouse half a mile from downtown with an upstairs bedroom and bath. It would be available after renters found a new place. We were fortunate in our timing, and went ahead with that purchase while getting our old house ready to put on the market. It needed a lot of cleaning, repainting inside, trimming of trees, improvement of our driveway, and installation of a new septic system (the 1975 system would no longer pass code).

All that was accomplished in due order, but a bigger problem was what to do about our dog, Gent, a 13-year old Chesapeake Retriever we had had since a puppy. Such a loyal and good friend all these years, but there was no room in our new place for a dog. Another stroke of good fortune—through the Animal Shelter on the Island, we met Linda Howell, who takes in older dogs. She had three other dogs on her ten-acre place in the country, with a pond for Gent to swim in, and even an indoor couch that would be his very own. When Linda met Gent, they got along great, as he soon did with her other dogs.

Meanwhile, I diagrammed the floor plan of our new place in town trying to figure out what furniture to keep, and where to put it. The goal was to make our new home as comfortable and familiar as possible for Gene, and to keep all of the furniture, paintings and other things that she especially valued.

We had about two months to get ready for the move. We divided the task into four main categories—what we kept for the new place, what we would give to Good Will, what would go to Consignment Treasures on the Island, and what would go to the dumpster (before we were done, we filled six of them!). We also gave a few very old things to the San Juan Community Theater for use as props in some of their plays set in earlier years.

One funny story within this hectic process. For more than 25 years we had kept our son Cal's oars on the wall of our garage since his years at Stanford rowing on the crew. They were beautiful red and white maple oars, still in good condition. I called him to ask if he would like them, but his family didn't have room for them and he thought they would make good firewood. Next I called Ben, our oldest grandson, who was rowing crew for a Seattle high school. He also deferred, noting that oars these days are fiber glass, both lighter and stronger than maple. But we didn't cut them up. They now adorn the walls of the San Juan Island Yacht Club.

We were soon to find that moving to town would be an adventure but not fun and games.

Chapter 12

Moving to Town

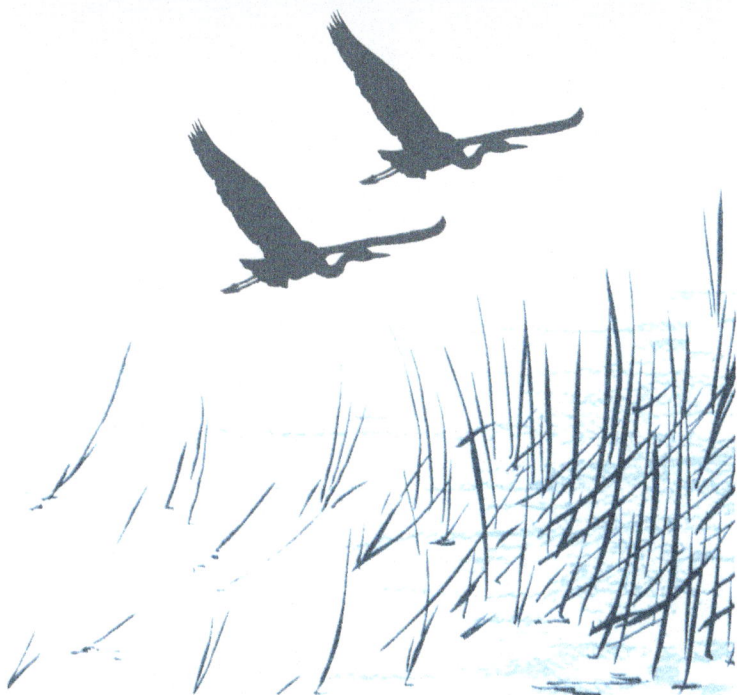

With about two months to prepare for the move, we had some breathing room. Gene and I visited the new place in town twice, even as the renters were still there, and made plans for what would go where. Gene liked the layout, but could not grapple with any details.

As we proceeded with all of the things to get the old house ready to put on the market, I also had to plan how to purchase the new town house. It was becoming clear that I needed to establish a guardianship for Gene, which would become part of how we listed ownership of the place in town. We planned to put the town house in my name, since Washington is a community property state anyway.

For a short time Gene and I tried to prepare for the move together. We brought in a dumpster as a way to start off-loading anything that we didn't want and was of no value to others. But it soon became obvious that Gene would not be much of a help. Dealing with our thousands of books was a good example. I would ask her to go through bookshelves and stack any books she didn't want on the floor. Then, if I also didn't want them, they would go to the garage in boxes awaiting removal to the Library's annual book sale or the dump. But that plan never worked. Gene would move stacks around, put some books elsewhere, and it was useless to start over.

About that time I read a book by Barry Peterson, *Jan's Story: Love Lost to the Long Goodbye of Alzheimer's*,[1] which helped me to decide to take charge of the move if we were to ever get it done. Returning to the book example, however, that was easier said than done! During the coming weeks, when I put boxes in the car (books labeled for the Library or elsewhere), they would pop up back in the house before I could drive away!

These excerpts from entries in my journal during just one week of those two months of transition give some idea of what I was up against.

January 3, 2011: *Attempts to segregate books by house, storage or dump don't work; categories get changed and all books end up on the floor. Hard to keep any order in the house. Though we both know the move will be therapeutic in the end, Gene is very agitated and confused about it. A larger dose of Zyprexa is decreasing delusions without any worrisome side effects, but Gene keeps asking me "Where will we sleep tonight?"*

January 6, 2011: *In morning, Gene was very worried where a favorite pot with a red cover went; "It must have been stolen by neighbors"; later we found it where she had put it in another room.*

January 8, 2011: *Questions in the middle of the night—"Where are we? Can we go home?"*

January 10, 2011: *Found our only salt and pepper shakers in a small sack of silver. Finding bird food upstairs where we always feed our cat. Also am finding surprising things in surprising places, such as unintelligible post-it notes all around the house, a suitcase packed with assorted items—clothes, silver, knives, jewelry, old pictures. I'll have to go through everything or we'll lose some treasures.*

We had excellent help come moving day in late February. An on-Island mover with a big truck and many years of experience, plus his niece who packaged everything up professionally. The new place had been well cleaned, and we moved all of the furniture we wanted into the rooms, and were able to sleep there the first night.

But the next days and weeks were very difficult. Gene was totally disoriented and upset. She kept asking, many times a day, "Where do we live?" and "Will we be here tomorrow?" On the other hand, it was interesting to note that she never looked back, and had forgotten the old house already.

The move for our cat was also a problem. Gene had always liked cats, and I hoped that would help with the move. But our cat became incontinent (both ways!), and after a week we found a new home for her (not a euphemism!).

So we accomplished the move as well as could be expected, but the next challenge was to get a lot more caregiver help. I was past denial of the stress building on me. Finding caregivers would supposedly be easier in town than where we had been, but I would soon find that Gene's accepting help would be another big challenge.

Chapter 13

Getting Help

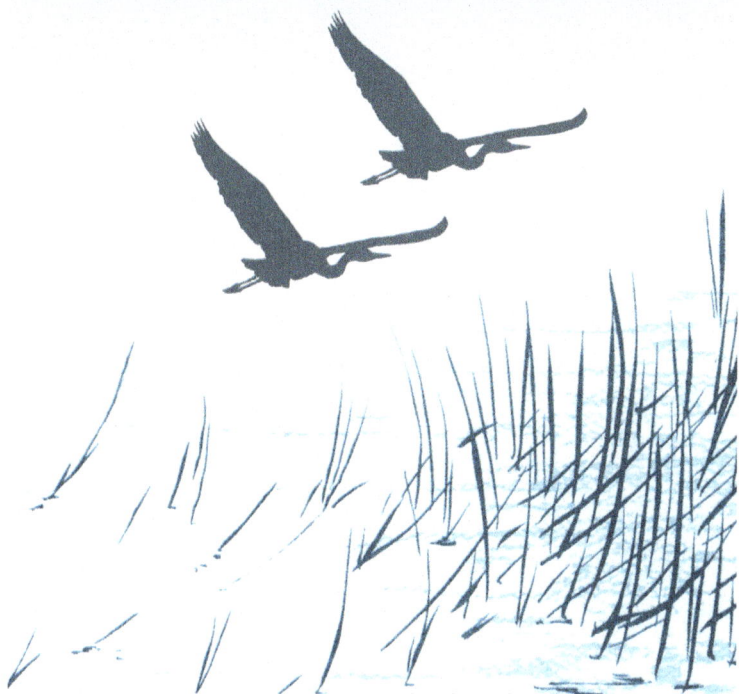

So we were now in town, getting settled into a smaller place. Some things were simpler, but the care problem was still a 24-hour challenge. The main challenge was to find caregiver help, sooner than later.

Gene was very confused, agitated, often angry at me as her closest target, and unable to do much on her own—a tough combination. My goals were to re-assess her medication, pull together a caregiver team in an effort to keep her at home all the way if possible, keep her in contact with people as much as she could handle, get regular exercise, and support each other in trying to simplify our lives with a regular structure and routine.

With updated advice from her family physician, the neurologist who had seen her for years, and a psychiatrist colleague at the University of Washington, we fine-tuned her medications in an attempt to reduce her agitation, anxiety, and continuing paranoia while still avoiding too much sedation.

I still wanted to avoid the nursing home if at all possible. Recall her claustrophobia from being caught alone in an elevator during college. She would never tolerate being confined in a locked facility. During the first weeks in our new town house, locks were already a big concern for her. She was either worried that people were breaking in and stealing things, or that she would get caught outside without a key to get back in the door. We set up a hidden, secret place to keep an outside key, but she could never remember where it was.

Next, I sought out advice from nurses and staff of the Senior Center about potential caregivers who could step in on a team basis, at first on a part-time basis.

Here are some representative entries from my journal that illustrate the challenge ahead of us.

March 16, 2011 (three weeks after our move to town): *Days blur (last three days seem like a month). Gene not doing well. Still can't grasp the concept that we have moved. Can't plan next 10 minutes. Loses her purse in the house every 15 minutes. Talks less, walks slower, mostly not angry, more in a daze. Doesn't know the day. Never remembers her pills. Putters around the kitchen. Can't make coffee anymore. Burns out coffee pots. Keeps wondering "What do I do now?" When asked what she wants to do, answers "I don't know." No animation anymore.*

Urgency to build a caregiving team is building. If we can't make it here, nursing home is the only other option. Assisted living place does not take Alzheimer's patients. If I break, it's 24-hour live-in care upstairs or the nursing home. (Later note: I was still under the illusion that a caregiver upstairs could handle our situation!).

March 22, 2011: *Meeting with Karen Antia (Later note: she would become our lead caregiver of a team of four others by the end of the year). Gene and Karen had known and liked each other for 15 years, and had served as co-presidents of the Garden Club. Gene very angry with me for "trying to push my friends on her." Karen very patient, calmly* *spent next two hours with Gene, ended up talking and hugging each other, plus agreement that Karen could help Gene with our garden and bird feeders. But Gene still very angry at me, no clue of my stress or utility.*

Later "conversation" about where we are, and what we need to do now. Avoid withdrawing from people (Gene's mother had been depressed, withdrawn and died at 75). Our joint goal to make it possible for Gene to live long-term in our new place, to stay here beyond my major illness or death. No understanding of all this, but didn't expect it. Initial anger and situation forgotten two hours later.

March 23, 2011: *Other caregivers on the team are now identified, but they have a 100-year old client and are not yet available. Another teapot burned out. Gene left gas on the stove, so will move it out and fill the hole with an electric stove. Finally got agreement that Gene won't try cooking anymore. Microwave with child lock is my territory, and we do fine with TV dinners plus salads that Gene makes.*

April 3, 2011: *Gas range went away yesterday while Gene was at the Library. New electric stove will have a red light if turned on. Gene says she will not use it. (Later note: but she did try a couple days later, touched a finger on a burner, so I removed all the knobs—and never found them again!)*

April 12, 2011: *Time passes quickly! Gene seems to have bonded with Karen (we call it companionship, not caregiving), though she usually can't remember* *her name (but always her smiling face). Karen now 15 hours a week, so Gene has a life (and me too!).*

But Alzheimer's gradually worse—lost her wedding ring, bought her a new gold ring. Everything now revolves around food, Gene eating all the time and gaining weight. Often can't figure out how to sequence hot water, filter and coffee.

April 22, 2011: *Interesting last ten days. We actually took a planned trip to the San Francisco Bay Area, where Gene spent her teenage and college years. It was clearly our last trip off the Island. Trip very confusing and disorienting.*

May 1, 2011: *At a family member's suggestion (and against my better judgment), Gene and I looked at a CNN special Unthinkable: The Alzheimer's Epidemic. It was well done, but as expected, full of how it only gets worse, has no cure, involves the whole brain as personalities fade away, and may end up not being able to talk or even walk. This was hardly therapeutic! What a mistake. We held hands, as usual, all the way through this long program. Especially poignant places, like the Long Goodbye, were painful to watch and hear. Not sure how much understanding Gene had, but am afraid that she already knew all this. We ended up agreeing that we were here for each other and doing everything possible to deal with all this (still including cuddles every night and dancing to music of the 50s, 60s and 70s).*

May 10, 2011: *Gene's new norm now is: get up in the morning, get dressed, make coffee (usually needs help), then nothing to do. Never knows the day, no concept of time, whether night or day. Often goes to bed in a dress. Can't get her to wear a night-gown. Gets dressed again in the middle of the night. Words jumbled together on many occasions, but not talking much anymore.*

May 17, 2011: *Main problem is how to occupy Gene during the day. After breakfast just sits down and stares out the window. Karen was off-Island for several days, but is back and Gene recognizes her less by name than by her face. Doesn't really read or watch TV. But she seemed to enjoy a Charlie Chaplin movie a few days ago. Sometimes says that she feels "funny in the head." Almost three months after our move, still sometimes asks "Where do we sleep tonight?"*

May 22, 2011: *Gene's acceptance of Karen's companionship is intermittent and unpredictable. Karen was scheduled today for a five-hour shift, but Gene wouldn't let her in the house. Neither Karen nor I could change her mind. She just gives me a cold hard stare, finally saying: "Don't bring your friends around and tell me what to do. Look at our neighbors. They don't need someone babysitting them. Why me? I've done OK myself all my life."*

In the aftermath of this kind of episode, I tried to mention that it is just a matter of time when we will need more help in the house, that we'll have to try to get used to it (mostly a one-way "conversation").

Despite all of these downers, occasional bright spots broke through our days, such as these:

- a five-hour time with Karen without angers and ending in hugs
- bringing me coffee and cookies in my study
- two short walks alone around the neighborhood without getting lost (I was watching).
- a Teddy bear sitting in my study chair
- very pleased with her new gold ring, even keeps it on during water aerobics in the pool

May 29, 2011: *The old house is selling, now in escrow. We accepted the first offer, a low bid, but we will still "come out whole." Glad to have its maintenance off our backs.*

Our next big task was to get more of a caregiving team together and establish a guardianship for Gene.

Chapter 14

The Last Nine Months

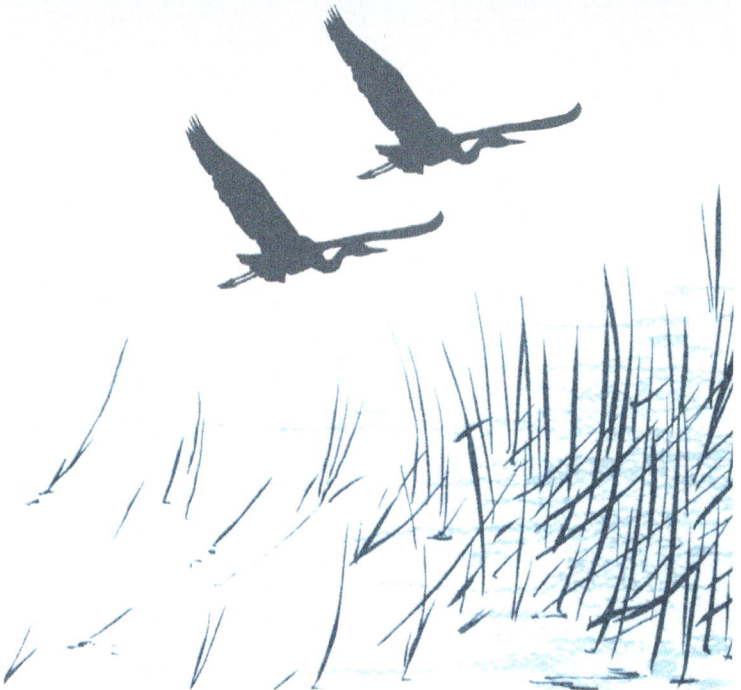

Assembling a caregiver team is much more difficult than one might imagine. Each caregiver has to be accepted and bond with Gene, they all have to work well together, and they have to be available. Fortunately, we have many excellent caregivers on the Island, but most have other clients and their own scheduling problems.

Through friends and word of mouth we were lucky to find Karen Antia as our lead caregiver. She had medical experience, including working with Alzheimer's patients. Within two months we had identified two other caregivers who had worked together before, but they were already fully scheduled. We gradually increased our coverage—12 hours a week at first, 40 hours a week six months later. But there are 168 hours in the week, and we were always behind the curve, as you will soon see.

Despite all of our efforts, Gene's course was ever downward over these last nine months, though with brief, relatively stable plateaus between events. She was often quite happy during much of this time, but angers and frustration naturally increasingly broke through.

I had been handling Gene's business affairs for years, and of course had her durable power of attorney for health care. But it was now clear that we needed to go through the official guardianship process to cover all of our business affairs going forward. We needed to consolidate and simplify our lives. With the old house in escrow, I worked with our attorney to establish the guardianship for Gene. This was a tough (and somewhat dehumaniz-

ing) process, involving appointment of a guardian ad lidem, who would meet with Gene to explain all the rights
she would lose— everything from voting to nine other
basic rights. The ad lidem person had to carefully exam-
ine our situation, assure that Gene's best interests would
be served by the guardianship, and prove in Court that she
was incapacitated.

I dreaded this process, especially if Gene would have
to go to Court herself and hear the Judge declare her per-
manently incapacitated. The appointed ad lidem person
was professional, highly skilled, sensitive and caring. It
appeared that Gene had very little understanding of this
situation.

At first she couldn't decide about going to Court herself, but finally felt she would rather not go to Court. So
the Judge reviewed the ad lidem's final report, and I went
to Court myself to hear the guardianship put in place for
Gene, the Incapacitated Person.

Meanwhile, Gene was having more and more problems, and the days and nights were getting longer. Everything became moment to moment. Being in town and in
our new place made it easier. My upstairs study kept me
at home almost all the time, and I could hear everything
that might be going on downstairs, including the opening
or closing of the front door.

Wandering and getting lost was our next challenge.
One late afternoon, after one of our better days, Gene said
something unintelligible, seemed happy and walked out
the front door. I thought she was looking for our neighbor's cat that we were taking care of during her trip off-
Island. So I waited a bit, and wasn't yet in the habit of
following her. But then I saw the cat and no Gene. I drove
all around the area, including downtown, and couldn't
find her. So I called the Sheriff's office to report her as

lost, and waited by the phone. Forty minutes later, I got a phone call from a woman who lived a mile away who had known Gene as an EMT. She had seen her on the road, looking lost, and brought her into her house to talk and call me. I rushed out there to pick Gene up, called the Sheriff that she was found, then tried to understand what had happened.

She wasn't angry, just confused, and no longer had *any* sense of direction or situational awareness. She had just walked out the door and turned right, kept walking along and turned in at the first place on the right in that direction. About that time, someone told me that Alzheimer's patients tend to turn to the right if they are right-handed. (That sounded interesting, but our own experience would later disprove it!)

So the next priority, of course, was to make sure that Gene had full identification with her at all times, even if she didn't have her purse. The California-based Medic Alert has many ways of doing this for patients with Alzheimer's as well as such other problems as seizure disorders. We put these labels in all of her clothes and shoes:

> Memory Impaired
> To Help: Gene
> Call: 1-888-572-8566
> ID# SR 298899

We also ordered a bracelet that would give her name, her problem, her medications, and people to call. (They also have pendants around the neck, but I knew that Gene would never wear one.)

When the bracelet arrived, Gene and I talked about how important it was, and I put it on her wrist. It had a special latch that could not be released by the patient, and I found it difficult to get on. But not surprisingly, the next day Gene wanted it off—*right now*!! "It's my body, my life, and I WILL get it off." If I wouldn't take it off, she would try to cut it off! Again she couldn't tolerate any restraints. So I took it off, called Medic Alert with the story and they told me that this was only the second time in thirty or forty years that this had happened; one man had cut his off with a hack saw! I thought of a GPS tracking device, but all of them would have the same problem—Gene would never accept one.

Not long afterward, the second wandering and getting lost happened. We had just finished dinner at a restaurant downtown, and had been talking with another couple at the next table. Gene was anxious to leave. Before I could pay our bill, she bolted for the door. It took me another twenty seconds to sign for my bill. By the time I could get to the door, she was gone! It was dark. She was nowhere in sight. After talking to the waitress in case she would return, I walked, then drove all around looking for her. No Gene. So another call to the Sheriff's office, and home to wait. Half an hour later, I got a call from the Bowling Alley. This time, she had turned *left* out the door and walked way up the main street to end up there. And again, she met a woman, another EMT, who knew her and called me.

Other incidents started to happen more frequently—surprises every day, as these examples illustrate:

- Becoming more fearful of being in a car; wants to open her door (while the car is moving) to get back home.
- Taking short walks outside all the time (mostly now with caregivers), but wants to turn back within a block, usually looking for me.
- Constantly worried that she won't have a key to get back in.

- Wandering unannounced to neighbors, sometimes inviting them to lunch when there wasn't any.
- Setting the table for six in the afternoon for a "dinner party" with nobody invited.
- Up several times a night, wandering in house as I worry that she will go outside; try to get her back to bed by turning off the lights; when that doesn't work, I turn the circuit breakers off as the only way to get her back to bed.
- Increasingly difficult for her to be in groups, even with close friends she had known for years; talked less, then as conversation left her would become angry and paranoid that they were talking about her.
- Thinking she would relate to and like the play *Little Women* at our Community Theater, we got tickets for a Sunday matinee; she seemed happy to go, but as soon as we sat down, she had to go home; I never knew why.

Over these months, we did develop a team approach to caregiving. The biggest challenge was how to occupy Gene, with her short attention span and frequent agitation. By now she could no longer read, and she could not do her volunteer job at her favorite place, the Library. We added medication to try to manage the agitation and ruled out a urinary tract infection, a common and often unrecognized cause of agitation in patients with Alzheimer's. And we started the supplement Melatonin in an effort to let her sleep better at night.

Each of our caregivers had her own special ways and skills to bring to Gene's care. Some were artists and brought out her drawing and painting interests. Often they could work together on puzzles (especially those with 50 pieces, not 500!), which became the most effective way to occupy her. Sometimes they could play together with puppets, listen to music, watch some movies (for a while, Charley Chaplin engaged her), or make such things as potholders.

Even as Gene became more dependent on me and the other caregivers, she would not know their names. Before any of them came, I would have to write down their names many times. In the mornings, she would open and close the front door time after time to see if the caregiver was there yet. Sometimes, even if things had gone well for a couple of hours, Gene would want the caregiver to leave. Other times they could do a whole shift and end up with hugs.

Some moments were especially poignant and painful:

- Trying to dress in the middle of the night and not being able to get her feet into a tote bag mistaken as pants.
- Going into our bedroom, shutting the door, and calling out for her Mother (who died twenty years ago).
- Telling me how sorry she is for me that she has Alzheimer's.
- Asking me during a cuddle in bed one night "What's wrong in my head? What am I to do? Will I get better?" What could I say to that except, "No, it won't get better, but I'm here with you all the way, as you were with me with my cancer 30 years ago and heart attack 11 years ago. Now it's my turn for you. Together we can cope with what happens." Then more hugs and cuddles. No other words.
- Not recognizing Cal, our second son, during his visit from Denver.

While trying not to admit it, all this was taking a greater toll on me. I was still not depressed, and was actually getting quite a bit of my own work done around the edges of Gene's care. There was so much to do. Here's a dream I had one night that seemed like a classic Alzheimer's dream:

I was in the back seat of a car driven by Gene at high speed down a narrow one-lane road toward a bridge; afraid of a crash; then the road stopped; Gene got out of the car; we're 100 feet over the water, with precipitous rocks below, let me drive the car and I'll try to turn around and we'll leave; instead Gene gets over a barrier, falls down rocks to the water; she can't get up; I can't get down.

Here's another sad turning point. Since Gene was getting up, often several times a night, getting dressed and sometimes trying to go outside, I decided on a fix. I went to the hardware store, got a door latch that she would not understand, and installed it on the inside at the top of the front door. That very night, she tried so hard to get out of the house, banging it so hard, that she pulled the seven-foot high door trim board from the wall, with many three-inch long nails protruding from the broken board!

This seemed like a nodal point. What to do? I decided this would be a good time to spend a night in the nursing home. After an hour, they found us a bed there (which turned out to be the hospice bed!). We drove there, against Gene's will, and got admitted. They put a cot in the room for me. Surprisingly, Gene slept quite well, but on awakening wanted out—RIGHT NOW!—and tried to get to the entrance. But it was locked, just as we feared. One of our caregivers soon came to take her home as I tried to mend fences at the nursing home. But this reinforced my worry that a nursing home would never work out for Gene. She would never tolerate locks or any restraints, and would require more ongoing sedation than I would ever want to put her through.

Despite this continued downhill course, there were bright spots along the way, when her basic warm personality shined through. No matter where she was, if she saw young children, she would light up and engage them in a happy way. When we were driving in a car, she would wave to people whether she knew them or not. She took to thanking me, many times, for what I did for her, telling me how much she loved me, with many hugs each day. She remained attuned to color, commented often about the colors of trees and flowers, and was always color coordinated in her own dress. On occasion, poppies from our garden would appear on our table, a Teddy bear would appear on my pillow, and the ultimate breakthrough—the buoyant, happy painting she did just three months before she died (page 157).

By early February 2012, it became clear that we needed caregivers seven days a week, 8 hours a day. Fortunately, we finally had a team of five very capable caregivers who were usually accepted by Gene and could deal with her mood swings. But things were getting worse fast. At times she would have a tirade against me and her life. "My life is bad, all is bad. Where is my Mother?" We had to increase the Zyprexa right up to doses just under toxic levels. I started to explore the idea (later proven impractical) of having a live-in caregiver move in upstairs. I also made an appointment with Gene's family physician to make the key decisions about future care options. We filled out Physician Orders for Life-Sustaining Treatment (POLST), including our specific preferences for antibiotics, intravenous hydration and tube-feeding in the event that treatment for her condition could no longer be effective. In effect, the POLST gives guidance for shifting from futile to comfort care.

Then, in mid-March, another nodal point. Despite medication, Gene was up and down all night. Neither of us got any sleep. She would dress, turn on the lights, walk around ready to go outside, and my circuit breaker trick no longer worked. She would just stay up, keep trying light switches that didn't work, and remain confused and agitated.

All this was not sustainable for either Gene or me. I wasn't getting any sleep, and my fatigue and stress levels were increasing. The only options seemed to be admission to the nursing home (which she would hate, and would require that she be so sedated that she would disappear as a person) or arrange 24/7 care at home. The answer was obvious, so we expanded our care team to five and planned for night shifts from 7 p.m. to 7 a.m.

This is when I finally realized that the upstairs bedroom for the caregiver would not work. The caregiver has to be in the same bedroom with the patient—and also cannot be in the same bed. So we brought in new twin beds downstairs and I moved upstairs to a different bed for the first time in 56 years. Even then the night caregiver got little sleep. Gene would talk a lot at night in bed, mostly unintelligibly, partly about babies and me. But Gene was prevented from walking outside or breaking her hip in the dark.

The POLST proved timely. Bad as things were, they would soon get much worse.

Chapter 15

The Last Week

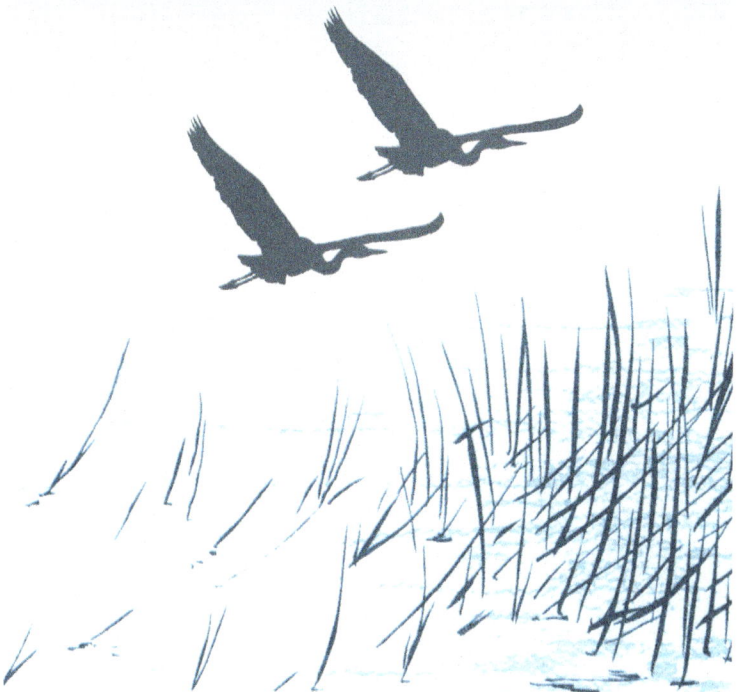

The last week started badly and went downhill faster than I could ever have imagined. We know that Alzheimer's is much more than a problem of memory and cognition, and that its end stages include impacts on such other functions as speech, mobility and reflexes. But I never expected, as I was soon to learn, that the ability to swallow could stop so quickly and with such devastating results.

Sunday.

Though Joan Byrne, the sleepover caregiver, last night told me that Gene talked much of the night, it was mostly unintelligible and probably in her sleep. This morning she awoke to a bad day. She dismissed the day's caregiver, so we spent two hours, holding hands, watching the great DVD *Echoes of Creation*, with its beautiful photography and soothing music. We had a close talk during that time renewing our commitment to each other and how we needed whatever additional caregiving help to make it possible to stay where we were. Then we were also fortunate to find a program with Bill Moyers interviewing Joseph Campbell about the power of myths, the meaning of life, and love as the source of life and essence of humanity.

Gene hugged often, had a slight dry cough, was not talking much, but was otherwise in no distress.

Monday.

Yesterday's slight cough was a bit more pronounced, but Gene had no fever, her lungs were clear, and she still was in no acute distress. She would cough with any sips of water or things like apple sauce, and started to avoid food or water. Her voice was less strong than usual. She remained affectionate, and hugged me often. As was so often the case, she was anxious who the caregiver would be today, looking outside often for her arrival.

Tuesday.

This morning was not good. She had some gurgling in the throat, spit out her oral pills, and refused any food or water. There wasn't any cough unless she tried to swallow. She didn't want to go to the Medical Center, but I insisted that we do. There, her lungs were still clear, the temperature was 100, and the chest x-ray unremarkable.

We went next door to the nursing home for a swallowing study by a speech therapist. No way did Gene want to go there, but we finally did. And no way would she swallow anything, but she finally swallowed once—abnormally.

We went home, but later that afternoon I wanted her seen again at the Medical Center and hospitalized for more definitive care. She was getting much more anxious. Who wouldn't be?! She knew very well that she couldn't swallow—a terrifying thought. We arranged to fly her off the Island to St. Joseph Hospital in Bellingham that evening.

So both of us flew that night to Bellingham in Island Air's fixed-wing medical evacuation airplane. With some of her former EMT colleagues assisting and with my aviation friend Bob Jamieson flying, Gene was well sedated and we had a comfortable flight to Bellingham, a trip that turned out to be her last.

Tuesday.

Arriving in the St. Joseph Hospital's Emergency Room at about midnight, so began what was to become an awful hospital course, in sharp contrast with the special care she would later receive in Hospice. We spent three hours in the E.R., during which time Gene was delirious and fighting restraints all the way. I gave her medical history and experience with past medications to the ER physician. She had been well sedated in the airplane with Ativan (Lorazepam). I was right there at the bedside the whole time, and kept asking for her to be better sedated. (Recall that she hates restraints of any kind!) All to no avail. Typical hustle and bustle of an E.R. with changing faces. She would keep looking at me and plead, "Help me!" And all I could do was ask for more sedation, still without success. I found that almost too painful to bear.

By now she had a low-grade temperature, a markedly elevated white blood count, and a chest x-ray showing right lower lobe pneumonia. The hospitalist physician came to see her, and I passed along a complete summary of her medical history. We reviewed her advance directive and the POLST. I agreed to IV fluids and a trial of antibiotics, at least this first time until her swallowing situation became more clear. He wrote orders for an MRI the next day to check out whether her dementia was due to Alzheimer's or multi-infarct dementia. He also wrote orders that continued her previous doses of Zyprexa, but without any interval sedation should that become necessary.

So upstairs we went to her hospital room at 2 a.m. They arranged for me to have a cot in her room. Gene was on IV fluids, antibiotics and in restraints. She was sedated at times, but kept waking up and trying to climb out of bed. It was always difficult to find the nurse and ask for more sedation. And if I did, she would have to check with the hospitalist, who was not readily available and a different physician every day.

Meanwhile, Gene kept crying, "Help me, and get me out of here!"—all too painful to hear. Instead of changing medication, the only change was to post a full-time, one-on-one attendant to sit next to her bed to make sure she didn't get out of bed and assist whenever a bedside commode was needed.

Wednesday.

Another swallowing study showed that she couldn't swallow. We cancelled the MRI. It would have been impossible with all her thrashing around. Nor would it make any difference what kind of dementia this was! She couldn't swallow!

I talked at length with two consultants, both excellent—Dr. Daniel Kizer, a geropsychiatrist who trained at the University of Washington, and Dr. Bree Johnston, a palliative care internist. At first, there seemed to be some chance, probably remote, that the larger doses of Zyprexa could be part of the swallowing problem. Tapering it down and bringing in an alternative medicine, Seroquil, might help, but it had to be given orally and might also do the same thing to swallowing. So Alzheimer's was almost certainly the cause of Gene's broken swallowing mechanism.

Although Gene's fever and white blood count were improving, her agitation and delirium in restraints continued whenever she was not fully sedated, which was at least one-third of the time. I kept trying to get her better sedated, but continued to be unsuccessful. "We'll check with the doctor," but nothing changed. I was there all the time, night and day, and got so tired and angry at hearing the bedside attendant keep repeating "I know, I know, just relax and lie back" whenever Gene kept trying to get out of bed.

Thursday.

This was pretty much a repeat of yesterday. Another swallowing study was no better—swallowing was now a thing of the past. Gene would never be able to swallow, and we could expect that she would keep aspirating. If she ever got out of the hospital, her future would have to be in a nursing home with a tube in her stomach. It was obvious by now that she would hate that, would pull out the tube at the first opportunity, it would get infected, and she would need restraints in a locked ward. For Gene and her independent spirit, that would be worse than a death sentence.

Since I would need to get a few things in order to stay longer in Bellingham, I flew back to Friday Harbor with a friend, picked up some things, including my cell phone charger, and flew my Cessna 180 back to Bellingham. I was very tired, but the flight went fine and the weather cooperated.

I was back at the hospital that afternoon. The situation was unchanged, and this was the last day that Gene recognized me.

Friday.

This was a terrible day. With Dr. Johnston, we reviewed in detail the options ahead of us. There were no good options. There was no effective treatment for Gene's problem. She had already suffered immensely, and it was time to shift to comfort care. We talked about options and locations of hospices. There were several in the area. The more we talked, I realized that we could never provide equivalent comfort care back home on the Island on this short notice.

The best option, which turned out to be superb for this situation, was the Whatcom Hospital Hospice, several miles south of Bellingham. This 12-bed hospice had been built by the hospital several years before. Together with Megan Crouse, a staff medical social worker, we made an extended visit to the facility. That was most impressive—very dedicated, caring and experienced staff and a beautiful facility in a pleasant wooded area. It takes an ecumenical approach to the best possible palliative care. They use no restraints at all, the beds are low to the floor so that no patient can fall out of bed and break a hip, they use no IVs or oral hydration (not even ice chips), and prepare a small subcutaneous site for infusion of morphine as needed to control any pain, agitation or anxiety. A very experienced nurse practitioner is constantly checking in on every patient, with a knowledge level of the end stages of respiration and life more extensive than any physician whom I have known.

There was a lot of paper work to complete before we could transfer Gene to the hospice. We scheduled the transfer for the next morning. Although Megan commuted each day to work from Lummi Island, she stayed in Bellingham that night so that we could sign all the papers first thing Saturday morning and complete the transfer that day. So kind and thoughtful of her. It was time to notify family of these new plans. Farthest away was Cal in Denver, who made reservations to fly to Seattle the next day and rent a car.

My feelings at the time were as positive as they could be under the circumstances. I felt no sense of abandonment. I was helping Gene to finally get some peace. It was what she would do for me, and the least I could do for her. I couldn't stand to watch her continue to suffer, and that was her only possible future. I was also feeling like the grieving goose I saw years before on a post of the Evergreen Bridge in Seattle for more than a week after his or her mate flew too low and hit a car.

Saturday.

After completing all the paperwork with Megan in the morning, I flew back to Friday Harbor to get pictures, stuffed animals, a quilt, music and other things that would give comfort and continuity to Gene in her hospice room if she ever woke up. I then flew back to Bellingham, getting to the hospice before Gene arrived. There was still enough time to get her room ready. There was also a long couch that would work fine as a bed for me. And Megan spent almost an hour talking with me about Gene's story, since this stage of her life (and our lives) was all about personhood and meaning.

Gene arrived by ambulance, well sedated, in the early afternoon. With great care, she was settled in to her room. There was a beautiful view out a large window, but she would never see it. She was asleep, in absolutely no discomfort, for the next (and her last) 24 hours.

It was unclear how long this stage would last, but we anticipated at least another day. By now all the family who might be able to come were on the way. We also invited Gene's caregivers on the Island to come the next morning if that were possible.

We know that people in coma or under surgical anesthesia can still hear, so we made an effort for one or more of us to be with Gene all the time, and to talk to her. Cal arrived in the afternoon, and we both spent time with her, then went out for dinner. We talked a lot about earlier happier times in the family to help offset this very sad time.

Sunday.

It was a long night. There was subdued light in the room, and the nurse practitioner checked in regularly. I listened to all of Gene's breathing, talked to her often, and knew that she was comfortable throughout. The dawn came early with birds singing at the feeders outside the window. With some nasal oxygen, Gene had good color and looked peaceful in the morning.

The rest of the family arrived later in the morning. They had their own special time with Gene. We played *Echoes of Creation* as background music throughout the morning. Karen, our lead caregiver on the Island, sang *Amazing Grace* in Gene's ear, and noticed a slight movement of her mouth in response.

That was to be the last response that any of us would see. Gene passed away quietly and peacefully in the early afternoon, and her long suffering was over.

Whatcom Hospice has two closing rituals after a patient passes. Family members are offered the opportunity to participate in a bathing of the body with lavender water (only I did that with a nurse). There is also a traditional ceremony about how patients enter and leave the Hospice. Since patients enter by the front door, they are to leave the same way. When the patient is ready to leave, three bells are struck and all caregivers assemble at the entrance for two minutes of silence in respect and caring for the departing person.

That last moment almost overwhelmed me. As she was wheeled out on the gurney, completely covered by beautiful blankets, and with the mortician's open vehicle waiting just outside the door, this was my last chance to see her. I peeled back the blankets from her face, gave her my last kisses, thanked her for all of her love, and said

"Thank you for being you. You are and always will be the love of my life. We are together forever."

After gathering up all of our belongings at the Hospice, and good talks with family, it was time to leave Bellingham. The weather was fine, but I was exhausted. Passing my self-check, I got in the airplane and flew back alone to the Island, with tears fogging my glasses all the way. But the Island is as nurturing for me as it has been for Gene. Entering the traffic pattern back at Friday Harbor, a pilot friend a few miles behind me already knew the situation and said on the radio, "Thinking of you, John."

PART III

Toward a New Future

I tramp a perpetual journey . . .
My right hand pointing to landscapes of
continents and the public road.

Not I, nor any one else can travel that road for
you
You must travel it for yourself.

It is not far, it is within reach,
Perhaps you have been on it since you were born
and did not know.
Perhaps it is everywhere on water and on land.

—Walt Whitman—*Song of Myself*

Chapter 16

An Empty House

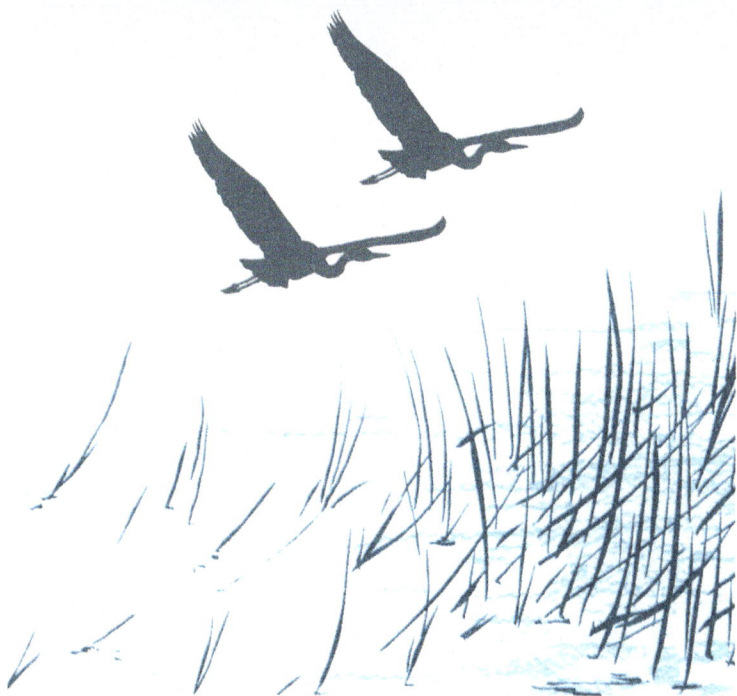

I was alone in an empty house, as most widows and widowers suddenly find themselves when they lose their spouse. Nobody to talk to or to care for. All of the remembrances of Gene throughout the house, just as she left them, but without any sound or movement to go with them. The loss of Gene, even though she had been disappearing for years, left an enormous void in my life.

I had always noticed that women who lose their husbands typically have the immediate and ongoing support of daughters, who provide help and companionship in the early stages of their loss. As the father of sons, each with busy lives of their own, this is not how it works. As is natural and good, they disburse back to their own lives and responsibilities.

The most striking change for me seemed to be the new dimension of time itself. I now had much more time than before—no caregiving activities that had dominated my life for years, no other schedules to keep except my own, all of the time structures and routines that Gene and I had developed over so many years now gone. It no longer made any difference whether I had meals at a certain time or any other things that we had done together as a couple.

What a different thing to shop for one in the market. It was much easier, quicker, and I could get only what I liked! But on the other hand it became such a mundane but necessary part of my life. As a non-cook, my only skill was with the microwave, so TV dinners, frozen veggies and fruit were the main items on my grocery list.

Despite all the new found time, there was plenty to do to fill it. The list seemed endless—notifications of banks, investment accounts, insurance companies, Medicare, Social Security, Medic Alert; notes to family and friends; arrangements with the funeral chapel and plans for the memorial service and celebration of life; and much more.

In addition to more time, the quiet of my new house was also a big thing to get used to. Although conversation gradually disappeared as Gene's Alzheimer's had advanced over the years, we still had some verbal connection and there was usually some sound in the house. I now found myself not only talking to Gene much of the time, but also to myself—and also answering myself! If I wasn't working at the desk, I would also play music more than before.

In rearranging the house, I moved my favorite pictures of Gene around so that there was at least one in every room. I kept many of her things as she had left them, such as on her dresser and on our dining room table. She would always have flowers on that table, so I continued that tradition. What to do with her many clothes was a big question. I ended up saving a few of her favorites, but getting rid of most to Good Will. I was trying to avoid making the house a shrine to Gene but keeping important remembrances of her in my daily life. It hurt to throw away things that were no longer needed, such as her pillbox.

On my first night back to the house, I still slept upstairs as the dance of musical beds continued. As you recall, I had moved twin beds in downstairs when Gene needed 24/7 care with a sleepover caregiver. My needs were now different. I wanted to move back downstairs and set up the old upstairs bedroom as an expanded study with a fold-up couch/bed. So my queen bed moved with me downstairs as the twin beds went away!

Our funeral chapel was on the mainland in Anacortes, Evans Funeral Chapel, which has served the San Juan Islands for more than two generations. I flew over there to make further arrangements for Gene. We had already decided on cremation, but there were still other details to complete. I picked out a nice brown companion box that would fit in on our mantle in the living room. It will hold both of our ashes, when mixed, after I go west. I could return to pick up the ashes in a couple of weeks.

Next on the list was the matter of burial. Our earlier plans for our ashes were to be in an urn under an oak tree, down the hill from our old house on the west side of the Island (with a great view of the Olympics and Vancouver Island!). This would no longer be possible. So I picked out a plot at the Valley Cemetery, a beautiful spot near the church where Matt and Amy were married back in 1991.

In planning for Gene's memorial service and celebration of life, I went through hundreds of old family pictures going back to her childhood. We made plans for these pictures to be sequenced with the *Echoes of Creation* DVD music during her service the next month at the Presbyterian Church.

Despite the solitude and loss over the first days and weeks in an empty house, there were some moments to laugh. When I went to hook up the electric stove again, I couldn't find the knobs I had hidden—anywhere! So I had to order some new ones to use the stove at all.

Then there was Gene's visitation that wasn't there. From the beginning I had talked to her and kept trying to listen or be sensitive to any messages she might have for me. I read more about the spirit world and visitations of spirits. One well-researched article by a physician in England in the 1970s reported that, among almost 300 widows and widowers, almost one-half had hallucinations or illusions of their dead spouse, especially after long marriages but usually not disclosed to relatives or friends.

One night I did hear a rustle elsewhere in the house, but couldn't find anything on getting up. But on another occasion during the day, I was sure this was the real thing. I was upstairs in my study, with nobody else in the house and the front door locked, when I heard and felt a strong presence, just outside my study. I was sure she would be on the stairs outside the door, walked out and instead heard steps on the roof. Instead of Gene, it was a friend who had agreed to fix a leaking gutter sometime; he had not wanted to bother me and just went up on the roof to do the repair!

Though I never saw or heard anything from Gene, as the time came closer for her celebration of life, I felt close to her in reliving so many memories of our times together in years past.

Chapter 17

The Memorial Service and Celebration of Life

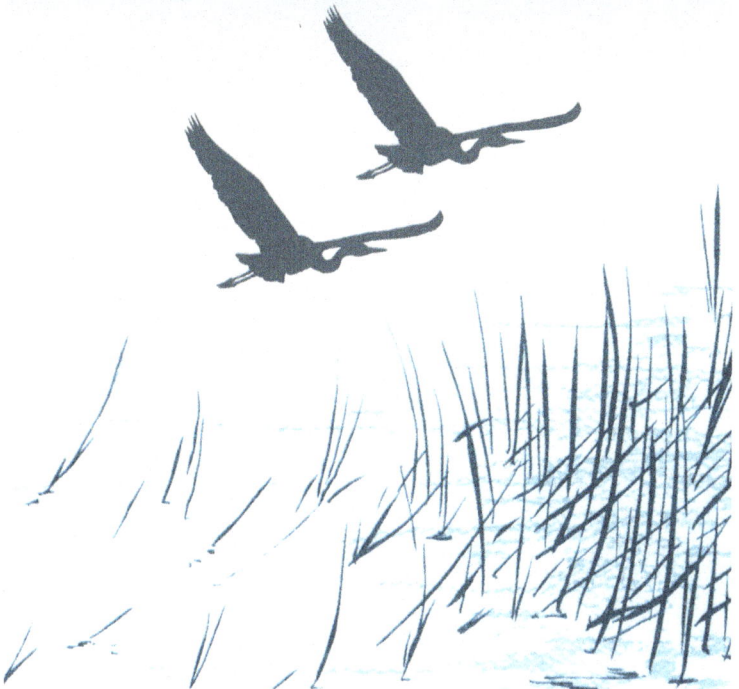

In keeping with Gene's life and spirit, I wanted the memorial service and celebration of life to be uplifting and positive. And they were. Held in the beautiful Friday Harbor Presbyterian Church on Saturday, April 28th, a day less than six weeks after Gene passed away, the entire occasion could not have been more memorable for family and friends who filled the church.

Pastor Joe Bettridge had been open and flexible from the start in making this a personalized tribute to Gene in her passage to the next world. She had always loved the 23rd Psalm and *Amazing Grace*, so they became an important part of the service. Together, we had always found inspiration and danced to John Denver's song, *The Eagle and the Hawk*, so that was also included. A sliding wall was folded back to make space available for the celebration of life immediately following the memorial service. The *Echoes of Creation* DVD was played and displayed in the Church, and later in that adjoining space. The pictures on the following page were on the front and back covers of the Church's announcement.

In Loving Memory
Eugenia (Gene) Deichler Geyman

February 9, 1935, ~ March 25, 2012

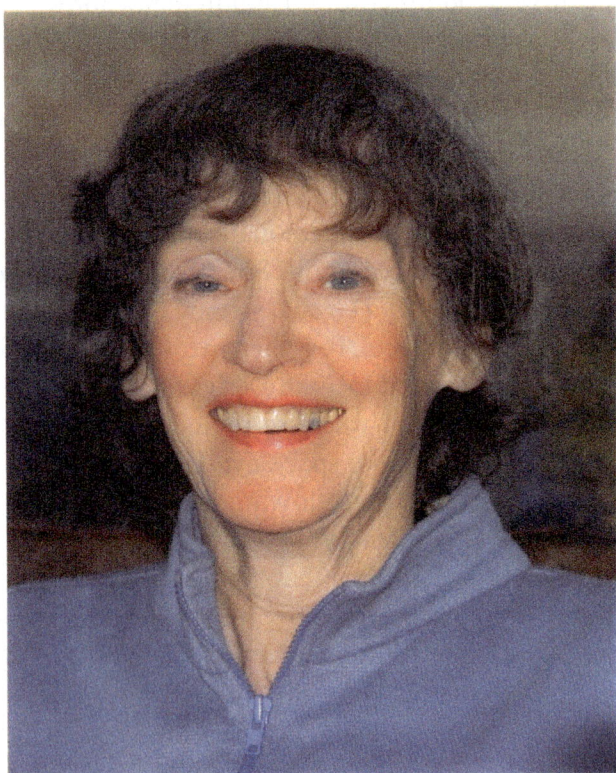

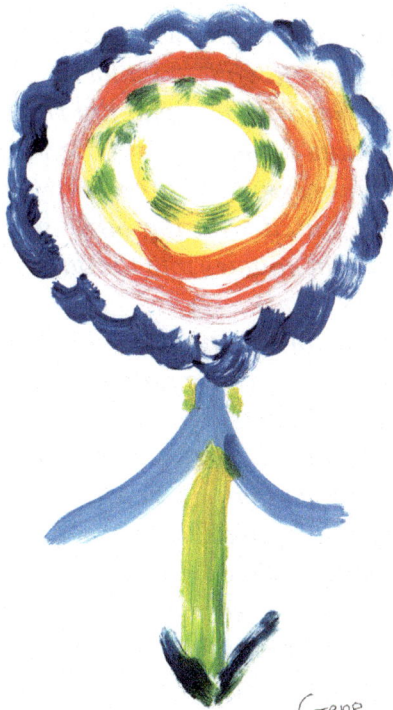

Painted by Gene - December 2011

The following eulogies and remembrances brought out the special personhood of Gene, the love of my life.

Here is what I said:

In one way or another, I have celebrated Gene's life every day since we first met in May 1955, almost 57 years ago to the day. This is a special day of remembrance for us all, but I will continue to celebrate her life every day as long as I live.

Our love story began when my sister, Carolyn Sabin (seated here), while a junior at UC Berkeley rooming with Gene in the Alpha Phi House, set up a blind double date for me and my friend, Jim, as we were getting processed out of the Navy at Treasure Island. I was paired with the other girl. We went ice-skating. Eight minutes into the date, we changed partners (sorry, Jim!).

We skated for a long time. I still know what Gene was wearing (a beige blouse with a tan and light green tweed skirt).

We dated for the next year as Gene completed her senior year and I finished premedical requirements (I'd been a Geology major in college). Gene supplemented her GI benefits from her dad's death on Okinawa (two months before the end of World War II) by reading to blind students. She had four marriage proposals at the time, including one from a young blind man she had read to over all four years in college. Remarkably, he ended up teaching high school in Los Banos, CA, also later marrying.

From the start, Gene and I had a marriage made in heaven. We always seemed to know what each other was thinking and could finish each other's sentences half way through. Over our 56 years of marriage, we grew and changed with each other, all the while supporting each other's changing interests and becoming closer, even after that relentless disease, Alzheimer's, joined us in the last 16 years. She sustained me through my cancer 30 years ago and heart attack 11 years ago, while I did the same for her with her Alzheimer's.

Words cannot express the depth of my love for Gene, but here is a start. She was a unique and special person, the best friend and soul mate I could ever hope to have on this earth. Always upbeat, with a warm and outgoing personality. Here are some of her traits:

- *she was smart: always able to cut through to the basic point, often before I could. Very good with words, a great reader of all kinds of things (English major) and filled with a zest for life.*
- *she was kind and caring: found the good in almost everyone she met, and they were the better for it.*
- *she was gentle but strong-willed: she was very direct, but never rude, and her gentle and independent spirit shined through.*
- *she was flexible and adaptable: enough to put up with me over the years and adapt to as many relocations as she had made growing up herself. (prior to our 22 years full-time here on the Island, 15 years in one place was the maximum for both of us).*
- *she was very much her own person and had an incisive sense of humor: one small example— we had two matching dressers that had been in her family. One was taller (mine, unfair*

159

since she had more clothes!) than the other. One day some years ago, she taped this message on mine: "**G.G to J.G.:** *Again: I trust you notice MY dresser is beautifully clean and well-ordered—whereas next to it is this very blankety-blank dresser.* "

- *she was creative and artistic: she was a gifted puppeteer, making all her hand puppets and creating her shows for children from old legends and stories. She was a very good writer, and wrote an excellent book, Ghost Pilot. A gifted teacher, she was well remembered by kids lucky enough to have her as their teacher in the primary grades.*

- *she was courageous and selfless: witness the grace she showed as her illness advanced and as she kept giving and caring for me and others as she could.*

So now, at this juncture in our journey: I give thanks to you, sweetheart, for being YOU through all these years, for your beautiful heart and soul, and for making my life better, as well as those of others fortunate enough to have known you. I am the luckiest person on the planet for having spent more than 56 years of my life with you. You have always been the light of my life. You have been, are, and always will be the center of my life. We have been as one, and will remain so. I take comfort every day in feeling you are still with me as we continue our dance of life. I rededicate to you my pure and unconditional love forever. Our ashes will go together to the Valley Cemetery of this beautiful Island (but let's not hurry that along!)

Our place will be just down the hill from the church where Matt and Amy (seated here) were married 21 years ago. There we will be able to fly up and around, at least on nice days; I assure my pilot friends at the airport that we will remain clear of the traffic pattern!

This is what Gene's brother, Clark, said:

My big sister Gene (or Bee as her family called her before she went to college) was, as I suppose are many big sisters (she was born two years before me in Atlanta), highly protective and supportive of her younger siblings, in this case me and our younger brother, Allan.

I recall Gene practicing her reading and writing skills on me when she was very young. She developed these skills during her first two years of grammar school in Virginia. The resulting advantage to me, because of my sister, was I could read and write before I entered kindergarten. She continued to help me socially and in school, when I asked, until we both ended up in the same University, but with different majors. She maintained her special literary skills throughout her life, as a teacher, mother, author and avid reader. I never met anyone who read as many books as my sister.

Our family moved many times because of our father's work as a structural engineer during the Depression and Gene had the unusual ability to make new friends and acquaintances whenever we relocated to a different city or state. She always included me in her new social network.

I have many memories of Gene but one stands

out above the others. While on vacation in Santa Cruz, California in 1945, Gene and I were awakened by our mother who was hysterical and in tears. Our mother, who had just received the dreaded WW II Department of Defense telegram, announced in a barely audible voice that our father had been killed on Okinawa. She left and both Gene and I were speechless. When we calmed down somewhat, we discussed what we should do next. I remember Gene telling me we should support our mother as best we could, look forward and not backward and carry on just as we knew our father would have wished us to do. I believe Gene maintained this attitude throughout her life and, especially, during her illness.

My sister, Carolyn Sabin, recalled:

As college roommates, Gene and I shared into the night discussions concerning the state of worlds, both large and small, unhampered by the youth of our actual experience. We were free and having fun. Gene's light touch and innate sense of humor made that year and those to follow special. I will miss being greeted in the way only Gene did, as . . . "dear girl."

We also heard some remarkable remembrances by some of Gene's caregivers in the late stages of her Alzheimer's. Here are three examples:

This from Karen Antia, her lead caregiver:

Gene always had a compliment on her tongue. Her smile could light up a room, and we spent much time laughing and sharing the good in life...

Later, even when she was unable to converse

162

as she once did, she made her feelings known up to the end. Her eyes were so expressive that you could read her thoughts and feelings if attentive. . . . Accomplishing tasks and completing anything was of great importance, as her life became smaller and her world more limited. She worked hard those last days being as independent as she possibly could.

Being with Gene was like returning to a simpler place in time and we both loved being in the world together. Our time was spent enjoying the important things in life, a beautiful view, sun on our faces, the wonder of God's creations and creatures of all sizes, the joy of walking barefoot in the sand, throwing pebbles to see them ripple. . . The last night we spent together when I said good night, Gene got out of bed, came around to my bed, gently kissed me on the cheek, and patted my shoulder, as if I was her little girl. She then returned to her bed and turned off the lamp. I softly said 'I love you, Gene, goodnight,' and she replied 'yes.' I will never forget that moment in time, Gene's sweet spirit, and I know we will meet again in another place and time.

This vignette from Susan Campbell Webster, an artist and one of Gene's caregivers in the last months:

Little more than a week before Gene's death (and she was so radiant and physically energetic that you never would have thought that death was imminent), I wanted to try to get her to let me help wash her hair. Gene was mostly reluctant to be helped. She seemed to feel she ought to do things herself. Her spirit of self-reliance was always the wall her caregiver gals had to get over. We were at

163

the dining table puttering around with coloring and painting and I suddenly began printing out with heavy pencil what I was saying to her and holding it up for her to read. Lots of times she couldn't seem to read at all so I made sure the printing was big and very legible. She seemed quite riveted by it and began carefully saying the words. I wrote that we should wash her hair today. She read it back to me, nodded and began taking her blouse off! I was so surprised and hardly ready for this adventure. Immediately we went into the bathroom, I found the shampoo and we began. It was easy, and Gene was very appreciative! That was the thing. Once she decided she was going to do something—with my help—she was so thankful. . . . There was no question how she felt. She was adorable. So full of love and thanks. Those times just made my whole day and lingered with me even after I got home.

After we washed and dried her hair and arranged it—very important: the arrangement of the bangs and sides—we went back to the dining room and I thought to continue the winning streak with more printing. I began printing the alphabet and Gene began singing the tune we all learned in 1st grade. We sang it together and then she took a piece of paper and sang and printed perfectly the entire alphabet until the U, faltering just a bit at the end and needing my help to finish. I was amazed.

And this from another of Gene's caregivers, Nancy Wilson:

When Gene and I were on a walk in town, she would often link her arm in mine, or take my hand and swing our arms—it felt so innocent and fun!

This from Jean Dowling, a long-time friend living on

Orcas Island:

It never occurred to Gene how beautiful she was. Her focus was outside of herself toward her family and many friends. What a gal.

And Nedell Crawford, a long-time friend on the Island, added:

Gene leaves so many of us with endearing memories of her marvelous energies, her kind and gentle ways, and her truly magical smile. She was truly a beautiful Lady in every sense of the word!

And this from Kathy Chadwick, a fellow walker of the Friday Walkers:

Gene always brightened when she saw me and made me feel welcome and accepted. She was the sheen in the fabric of my sense of community here.

As but some of many examples, all of these remembrances paint a very clear and consistent picture of the marvelous human being that Gene was and her spirit that lives on in the lives and hearts of those of us fortunate enough to have known her. She showed us how to live—and to die—and her gallant spirit lives on.

After the Church service, the celebration of Gene's life really was a celebration. Travis Potter, an Island paramedic, played the bagpipes. Gene's service as an EMT was honored by Emergency Medical Services. And her puppets were there in a display put together by the San Juan Island Public Library. The entire occasion was uplifting, remaining true to Gene's lifelong spirit.

Chapter 18

Bereavement

Where am I?
Who am I?
How did I come to be here?
What is this thing called the world?
Why was I not consulted?
And if I am compelled to take part in it,
Where is the director?
I want to see him.

—Soren Kirkegaard

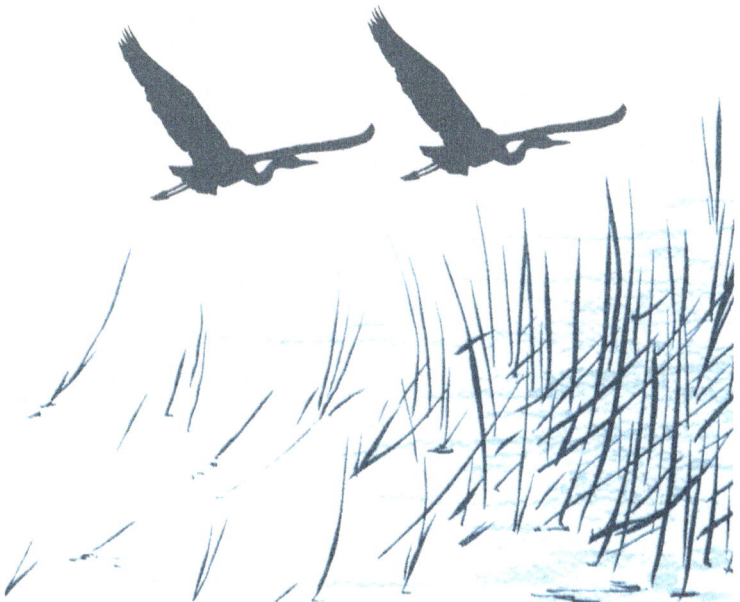

As everyone knows who has gone through the grieving process, it is hard—really hard. We all grieve in different ways and for different periods of time. And as they say "You never get over it, you just get used to it."

As Dr. Tom Holmes, psychiatrist at the University of Washington, recognized in the 1970s, loss of a spouse is the highest stress level of any that can befall us. That is especially true after a long, close marriage. And we also know that the surviving spouse frequently doesn't live more than six months beyond the death of their spouse, entering a depression without recovery.

I had been grieving in my own way for many years during Gene's last years as her Alzheimer's advanced. But even then I was not well prepared for the finality of her passing. All of a sudden, there was a gaping hole in the structure and rhythm of my life. In many ways, the task was to start over and put it back together a new way.

My feelings were mixed. On the one hand, I was glad that Gene no longer had to suffer, and that she was in a better place, wherever that is. And I was relieved of the day-to-day, even moment-to-moment worry and stress of her care. But the enormity of her loss filled my days and nights, aggravated by the silence of the house I remained in. Despite her illness for so long, I missed her companionship, caring, voice, spirit, and enveloping love.

While I kept busy during the days, nights became long and lonely, and sleep was a problem at first. I avoided sleeping pills, but Melatonin was often helpful.

Loneliness was my biggest problem, especially when the phone rang less and the condolence cards stopped coming. I was aware that my loneliness was situational, in the aftermath of Gene's death, and that the thing to avoid was its becoming chronic.

As all surviving spouses soon find, I had to rebuild my life and carry on. Gene would have pushed me to do that, and be disappointed if I couldn't do it. As Kirkegaard said more than 150 years ago, the process of bereavement calls into question our personal identities. That was not a problem for me. I had plenty of ongoing and satisfying work in my research and writing on health care, together with supportive colleagues and friends in the Island community and elsewhere. There was no shortage of interests and things to do. The task now became sorting out the most meaningful ones with a shorter time horizon than I had used in earlier years. I was fortunate to be in good health, still active, with the motivation to pursue present and new future directions.

These are some of the heartfelt feelings from our friends that I treasured and found especially helpful in accepting Gene's loss and gaining confidence to move on into a new life.

From one of her caregivers in her last months:

I'm happy Gene has gone. I need not say why and I know you do not think I am hard hearted to say it. She deserved to have her suffering, anxiety and regret end. And you deserve to have a bit of peace—though I can only imagine how much you will miss the loveliness that was the heart of your Gene and which shone out from her always . . .

From one of her EMT colleagues, who had been

through the loss of her husband after a long and close marriage:

My heart bleeds for your loss, but I know that Gene is with you and she has her total faculties and is watching over you now. Wrap yourself tightly in the good and loving memories. I wish I had some true words of comfort, but there are no words to fill the gaping space.

From a friend since our first years on the Island, who had lost her husband several years earlier:

Your love for Gene was the most wonderful gift you could have given her, and I know you filled her heart with joy as she did yours. As you remember the many special times you shared in your life together, I hope they will bring smiles to your heart.

This from Megan Crouse, the medical social worker who went out of her way to get to know and support Gene and me during our hospice experience:

It was glorious to witness your love for Gene, each moment to the end. Keep writing!

Even my male friends could be articulate. This from a classmate in medical school more than 50 years ago, a former Marine, who had also lost his wife after a long marriage:

Gene was very unique—smart, creative, insightful, funny and very human—truly one of a kind. I'll miss our 'bookish' conversations. We'll struggle through—because we have to.

This from a physician friend since our years in residency training 50 years ago:

I can't imagine words that adequately describe the loss of your lifelong soul mate. We remember her as a unique person gifted in many ways— intelligent, artistic, an original deep thinker and Jungian admirer. You were so well matched in a complementary way which led to your closeness, each pursuing your own passion and yet shared values and interests. Your care of Gene was a labor of love but I'm sure difficult at times for which I hold you in great admiration.

This from a friend at the Fitness Center who sometimes took my money (not much!) in neighborhood poker games:

She was the light of your life . . . and you were there when she needed you most. My love and admiration.

This was not just a loss, but an opportunity to re-explore myself and build a new future. I started reading more widely than before into areas with a more spiritual dimension. Jerry Sittser's book, *A Grace Disguised: How the Soul Grows Through Loss*, was especially timely and helpful to me. As a professor of religion at Whitworth College with a master in divinity degree and a doctorate in history from the University of Chicago, he had lost three members of his family—his mother, wife and young daughter— in a tragic car accident when they were hit by a drunk driver. Three generations gone in an instant. His book is a must-read for all of us who have undergone major loss in our lives. His realistic but hopeful insights fill this fine book. These examples resonate with where I have found myself:

Loss is as much a part of normal life as birth, for as surely as we are born into this world we suffer loss before we leave it. It is not, therefore, the experience of loss that becomes the defining moment of our lives, for that is as inevitable as death, which is the last loss awaiting us all. It is how we respond to loss that matters. That response will largely determine the quality, the direction, and the impact of our lives.[1]

And further:

Catastrophic loss by definition precludes recovery. It will transform us or destroy us, but it will never leave us the same. There is no going back to the past, which is gone forever, only going ahead to the future, which has yet to be discovered.[2]

This observation by C. S. Lewis also resonated with me:

Bereavement is a universal and integral part of our experience of love. It follows marriage as normally as marriage follows courtship or as autumn follows summer. It is not a truncation of the process but one of its phases; not the interruption of the dance, but the next figure.[3]

There was never any question about where to live. Gene and I had made a one-way trip to Friday Harbor and San Juan Island more than 22 years ago, attracted by its charm, history and sense of community. We had found the community just as open and nurturing as we had hoped, and weren't about to leave it for another place where we would have to start all over in building a support system in our later years.

Soon after Gene passed, the Presbyterian Church planned a small group grief session for several people who had recently lost their spouse. As a long-standing non-church attendee who was more like a Unitarian who doesn't go to church, I surprised myself by going. I found it helpful to share my candid emotions with others confronting the same problem. I further surprised myself by starting to attend church and participating in a series of eight sessions along the theme of developing emotionally healthy spirituality, all led by Pastor Joe Bettridge and his wife Becce. Here again I found these sessions challenging but helpful in slowing down, surrendering my ego, simplifying my life, and accepting guidance from a higher power in rethinking my new directions. I was becoming more contemplative and honest with myself as to what my most important priorities will be for the remainder of my life.

I had not kept a diary for the first three months after Gene died. Here are some entries from my journal at that stage of bereavement:

At first, and still, I have made the house something of a shrine to Gene—her painting next to her ashes, pictures, the puppets, her favorite clothes, flowers on the table just as she always did. But now I'm realizing that I can't live in the past. I have to build a new future, but hopefully not alone. One can say that we're never alone, but those are empty words a lot of the time, especially at night!

So new chapters for us all with such a great loss. Uncharted territory. I'm sleeping lightly, often meditating peacefully at night re what next. The thing I've already learned is that I don't want to live alone the rest of my life. I need to share life closely with another person—a woman. Right now I'm in a male world, and miss the closeness, conversation, sharing and caring that Gene showed me how to do. Nobody can be just like her, but I now know that I can be open to starting a new relationship. Gene brought up that conversation many times in her last few years, and I know she would want me to do just that. Interesting how she sensed so long ago that she would die first.

Another important part of my "grief work" was buying an open-cockpit Curtiss Wright Junior, a 1931 design (the same year I was born) built from plans in Seattle in the early 1960s. Aviation and flying had always been my "spirit world" since childhood, and I still thought of myself as that kid inside. After concluding the purchase on e-bay, part of my next chapter became concrete over the next two months. How can you get depressed when you have to travel across the country to Delaware, package it

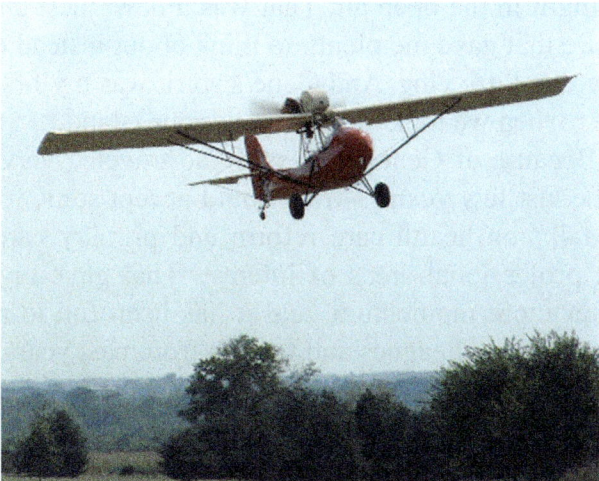

Another United Flying Octogenarian (UFO), the Curtiss Wright Junior

up in a Penske truck, and drive it back to the Island with another flying friend, Jonathan Taylor?

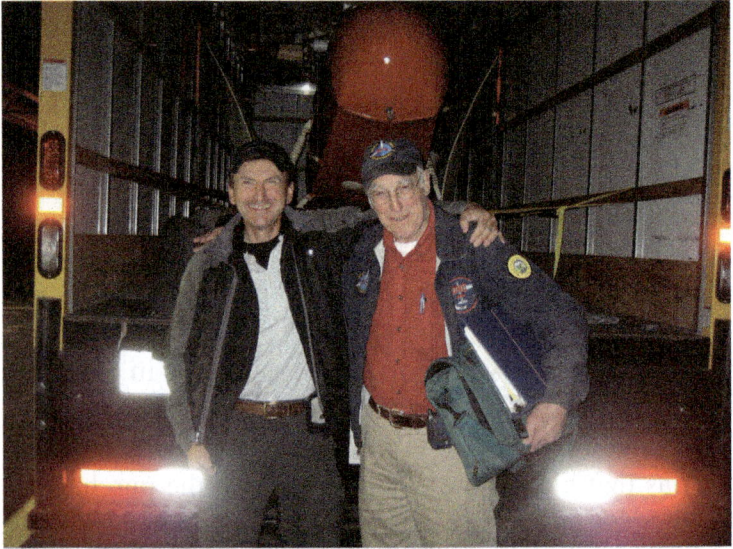

All the anticipation of the trip, the transport, and the first flight in the open air. That was a new quest and adventure that gave me plenty to think about instead of sitting around grieving. And Gene's spirit was my first passenger when we took to the air over our Island.

Because of Gene's illness, I had traveled very little for the last few years. Now I could accept some trips to give talks on health care reform and primary care, my main professional areas of interest. That gave my new chapter more momentum, and it has been fun to renew contact with colleagues and friends from past years.

Here are some entries in my journal six months after Gene's passing:

Working on this book has been therapeutic for me. It is my own way of searching for meaning in the trajectory of our lives together. And in reliving so many of our memories together, it does increase their meaning. I am now at peace, finding the Church sessions in emotionally healthy spiritualism helpful, sleeping better, and still not depressed. Already enjoying a slower rhythm and living more in the moment. Glad to survive the six-month marker for surviving spouses.

Am starting to think of possible new women friends. Had virtually never dated (high school and college had not been co-ed; nor was the Navy!). So the prospect of dating is daunting. So many things that would have to be symmetrical or complementary for two people at these ages to become a match.

Of course, in the best of worlds I could never replace Gene, nor would I want to. Our spirits are as one forever. People talk about closure. That's not what I want, but I do need to move on into a new and different chapter. Next are some of the things that I've already learned on this journey.

CHAPTER 19

What I Have Learned

Even the saddest things can become, once we have made peace with them, a source of wisdom and strength for the journey that still lies ahead. —Frederick Buechner

All we have to decide is what to do with the time that is given to us. —J. R. R. Tolkien

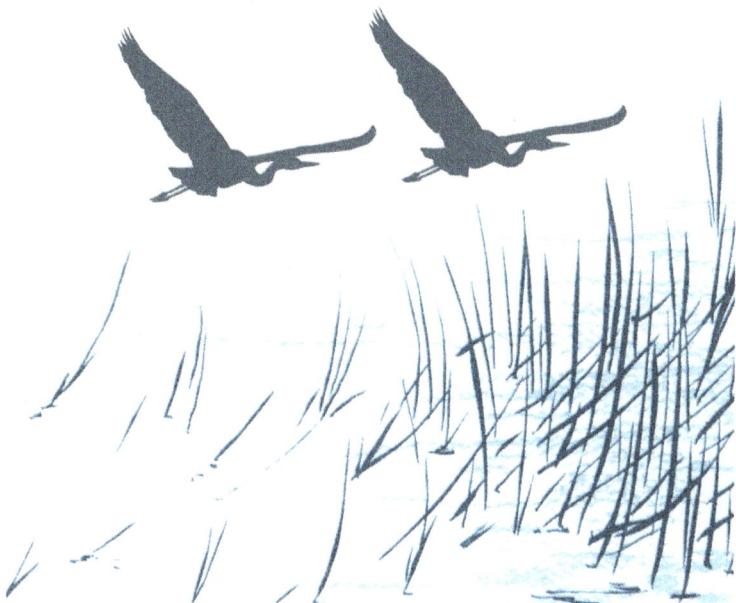

As **Jerry Sittser notes** in his excellent book, *A Grace Disguised: How the Soul Grows Through Loss*, the loss of a family member brings a sudden halt to business as usual. Time stops as we are forced to deal with the loss—not just a good time to reflect on the meaning of it all, but an absolutely necessary one.

There is much to be learned from Gene's and my experience with Alzheimer's. Much of what we could learn was only in retrospect. At this stage seven months after her passing, these are the twelve major lessons that I have carried away from our lives before, during and after Gene's struggle with Alzheimer's.

1. No matter what confronted us in dealing with Alzheimer's, the Great Thief of personhood, love transcends all.

Gene gave me a treasure trove of love, enough for five lifetimes, which I will savor for the rest of my life. That's who she was—looking outside of herself to others and the world, ever with a positive and caring approach. Even after her disease brought new limits, she kept finding new ways to show her love. In later years, as aphasia progressed with loss of words and conversation, there were still hugs, which she gave me many times a day, often with thanks for staying with her. We were both grateful to each other for our long, close and special marriage. As Joseph Campbell says in his book, *The Power of*

Myth, "marriage is the symbolic recognition of our identity—two aspects of the same being."

I was fortunate later to watch an interview of Joseph Campbell by Bill Moyers, during which he further described love as the essence of life, the great source of life, and the essence of humanity.

I have also found this poem by Guiraut de Borneilh (circa 1138-1200?)[1] helpful in understanding the full power of love:

So through the eyes love attains the heart:
For the eyes are the scouts of the heart.
And the eyes go reconnoitering
For what it would please the heart to possess.
And when they are in full accord
And firm, all three, in the one resolve,
At that time, perfect love is born
From what the eyes have made welcome to the heart.
Not otherwise can love either be born or have
  commencement
Than by this birth and commencement moved by
  inclination.

By the grace and by command
Of these three, and from their pleasure,
Love is born, who its fair hope
Goes comforting her friends.
For as all true lovers
Know, love is perfect kindness,
Which is born—there is no doubt—from the heart
  and eyes.
The eyes make it blossom; the heart matures it:
Love, which is the fruit of their very seed.

2. The narrative of the patient's story has to be understood and used as a guide to his/her care.

Especially when it comes to major illnesses in our later years, we need to incorporate the patient's life narrative and prospects of future quality of life into decisions about medical care. This frequently gets overlooked in our everyday quest to apply yet one more "magical fix" of technology that disregards what the patient might really want. Unfortunately, in today's medical world, driven more by tests and procedures than by talking, listening and understanding, there is little opportunity for physicians and patients to communicate enough in this area. To our detriment, more than we would like, health care has devolved to strangers taking care of strangers compared to the more continuous and closer physician-patient relationships in previous generations.

As you have seen in Gene'e life story, her elevator experience during college led to claustrophobia in later years that made use of any restraints beyond threatening. She was delirious in fighting restraints in the Emergency Room and hospital during her last week whenever she was not sedated. Suffering of the worst kind, and could have been prevented. And as you have seen, even when I as a physician and her husband was there throughout her ordeal, my advocacy often fell short of her needs.

3. Alzheimer's is more than a memory problem; it is a neurological disease with varied and serious impacts.

Although Alzheimer's disease is widely perceived as mainly a problem of declining memory, it is much, much more. It is a multi-faceted neurological disease, still poorly understood in its development, which can be treated but not cured. Its course varies widely from patient to patient. Problems that commonly become associated with Alzheimer's as it progresses range from problems of mobility, balance, posture and gait to swallowing, speech, tremor and behavioral changes. Patients typically become confused and disoriented, with many becoming angry and paranoid. Because of these kinds of associated problems, patients in late stages of the disease often require custodial care in nursing homes with 24/7 care. Although I had not previously seen inability to swallow as the final terminal event in Alzheimer's patients, I now understand that it is more common than I had thought, especially as a cause of recurrent aspiration pneumonias.

Unfortunately, Alzheimer's is increasingly common in this country as our population ages. There are now some 5.4 million Americans with the disease, a number that is expected to reach 13 million by 2050.[2]

4. As the disease progresses, it is difficult if not impossible to plan for all the contingencies ahead.

My original hope was that we could stay in our house of 21 years on the west side of San Juan Island all the days of our lives, adding caregivers upstairs as needed along the way. That hope turned out to be a naive hope at best. There was no way that we could predict the rate and kind of changes that we would experience as Gene's Alzheimer's progressed. As for additional caregivers, as one example, how could we have predicted what kind of care would be needed, when and where until her condition declared itself more clearly?

If you find yourself faced with the care of a family member with Alzheimer's, you can be sure that you will need increasing help along the way. But you are not alone. Your nearest chapter of the Alzheimer's Association can help you find what resources might be available in your community and region, such as adult care centers and support groups. In addition, your local senior center may put you in touch with various home-based care services.

5. Never give up, just adapt and re-adapt to changing needs of the patient and caregivers.

Throughout Gene's care, I kept telling myself to be patient, never to show disappointment, and always to be supportive no matter what was going on. Even when it didn't work out, I kept trying to adapt to changing circumstances, stay as flexible as possible, and even be creative at times. You learn to do things that you would never read in books. When she was sundowning, getting up at night trying to get outside at the risk of getting lost, I was proud of my scheme of turning off the circuit breakers when she wouldn't go back to bed—but only until it didn't work anymore!

6. While Alzheimer's is a relentlessly progressive disease, plateaus and breakthroughs happen and need to be nurtured.

While we know that Alzheimer's will only progress, we don't know the timing or rate of change. Plateaus can happen for many months or longer, and we need to treasure them as much as we can before the next downslide happens. And even as the disease advances, we can be surprised to see breakthroughs of insight and talents that we would never have expected. One example of Gene's insight being surprising was her wanting to talk, on many occasions over the last five years, of what I should do after she died. As for remarkable talent when she could no longer read, watch a movie, or talk clearly, witness her amazing painting (p.157) painted just three months before she died! How full of grace Gene was as her decline accelerated, in smiling at people, seeking out children, seeing beauty in trees and flowers, never complaining, and giving, giving, giving . . .

Sometimes Alzheimer's patients will come up with mystical and difficult to understand responses to questions. In his book, *The Caregiver: A Life with Alzheimer's*, Aaron Alterra (a pseudonym) describes his wife's response to his question of how she could account for her new gift of sleep? Her distinct response was "It plays on a different reed."[3]

7. Stay at home all the way, if at all possible.

In the last stages of Alzheimer's, the patient's world contracts to just what is immediately about. As life becomes a struggle to know what's going on, patients become increasingly confused and disoriented. So the more their surroundings can be familiar and give continuity to their former lives, the better. We kept trying to have Gene's favorite pictures, paintings, furniture, puppets and other things right around her at home. Change of location is usually threatening and disorienting when familiar surroundings are no longer there.

8. Shift from "curative" to comfort care as soon as further treatment becomes futile, taking into account the patient's desires.

It takes much more than a living will or advance directive Do Not Resuscitate order to provide the best possible quality of life and least suffering for patients in the last stages of Alzheimer's disease. Most hospitals remain more oriented to "curative" care than comfort care. They also have incentives to continue treatment beyond times that would help the patient. I was prepared for Gene's last hospitalization by having completed a POLST (Physician Orders for Life-Sustaining Treatment), and that helped to guide her terminal care. When further care appears to be futile, the POLST helps to shift to comfort care in hospice by asking the patient's guardian or person holding the durable power of attorney for health care to make decisions about tracheal intubation, mechanical airway ventilation, use of antibiotics, and artificially administered nutrition.

9. Reach out to family, friends and the community during care to build a support system for the patient and primary caregiver.

Both the patient and the primary caregiver do a lot better if they accept their lot and reach out to other members of the family, friends and whatever resources in the community might be available. Unfortunately, many patients feel a stigma in admitting their problems. Many caregivers then aggravate the situation by isolating themselves. In so doing, they place themselves at great risk of becoming depressed, less able to function, and their own premature mortality.

10. As the main caregiver, take care of yourself!

Despite the growing stress and work load of your caregiving role, try to get enough sleep, enough help, and stay engaged with your own life. Friends will help a lot, and you will hear more stories every day of relatives of friends fighting similar battles with the disease. Find ways to laugh when they come up, as I did for instance, when losing Gene in the market. (Not yet a time to call the Sheriff—I always did find her!). Remember that your loved one will be much worse off, immediately, without you.

11. Treasure your years and time together.

We need to be grateful for every day and year together. I found it helpful to assemble pictures on both sides of our family back to our childhoods. That ended up as a priceless treasure for me and our families. My great regret, however, was not having a record of Gene's voice. I had never thought about that, as almost all my friends whom I've talked to also admit. Except for several short clips of her voice on Cal's camcorder a few years earlier, we have no record of her voice.

12. Death is not the end!

As I became just one more among survivors of loss of a loved one, as happens some 150,000 times a day on our planet, I had no firm religious faith in the hereafter. By nature I have tended to need solid evidence for it. On the other hand, I have always been in awe of the coordinated wonders of the natural world. And like Kirkegaard in the last chapter, I have often asked myself the big questions about who's in charge here and what does it all mean?

After Gene passed, I have tried to be sensitive and listen for any messages that she might send me, and of course have wondered where her spirit has gone. Without any firm religious view about the afterlife, I have always been troubled by how varied and contentious the world's religions have been on the subject, even to the point of recurrent wars over conflicting views throughout history. But this statement by the surviving son after his mother's death resonates with me:

My mother was Jewish, my father an atheist, we went to Catholic school and attended Friends meeting. Each of these groups had a different view of where one went after death, but I know where my mother is—she is in me.

More reading and contemplation have not yet led me to any strong convictions about the afterlife, and obviously can only be minor scratches on the surface of a huge subject, but I have found some writings especially useful. Based upon wide experience as a hospice chaplain, psychotherapist, and thanatology researcher, Dianne Arcangel's 2005 book *Afterlife Encounters: Ordinary People, Extraordinary Experiences* presents the findings of her five-year international Afterlife Encounters Survey, including both data and stories for more than 800 respondents. She classifies the various types of afterlife encounters and reviews the world's literature on the subject.[4]

That gave me a more solid base upon which to rethink these questions, leading me to recall an incident in our own lives that I had long forgotten. In 1962, while we were living in Santa Rosa, Gene's mother visited us. While she and Gene were walking on the driveway back to our small house with a large window next to the front door, her mother suddenly said: "There he is!" She then described her dead husband, Gene's dad (who was killed on Okinawa in June 1945), dressed in white (whites were his Navy dress uniform). It was a visual apparition without sound, lasting perhaps half a minute. Though a skeptic on these matters, Gene's mother described it in detail. Gene did not see it, but told me about it then and many times later. All that increased my interest and wonder about souls—where they go, what they do.

Though it wouldn't have changed the outcome, I wish that I had learned some of these lessons earlier than later as Gene and I dealt with her advancing Alzheimer's. This last 16 years have been a journey, mostly in uncharted waters. But it's all part of our journey together. Each new development has brought new circumstances and new choices. The journey continues.

CHAPTER 20

Souls Walking On

What I once considered mutually exclusive—sorrow and joy, pain and pleasure, death and life—have become parts of a greater whole. My soul has been stretched.

—Jerry Sittser, theologian & author of *A Grace Disguised: How the Soul Grows Through Loss*[1]

To know the universe itself as a road, as many roads, as roads for traveling souls.

—Walt Whitman, *Song of the Open Road*

Life, so-called, is a short episode between two great mysteries.
—C. G. Jung

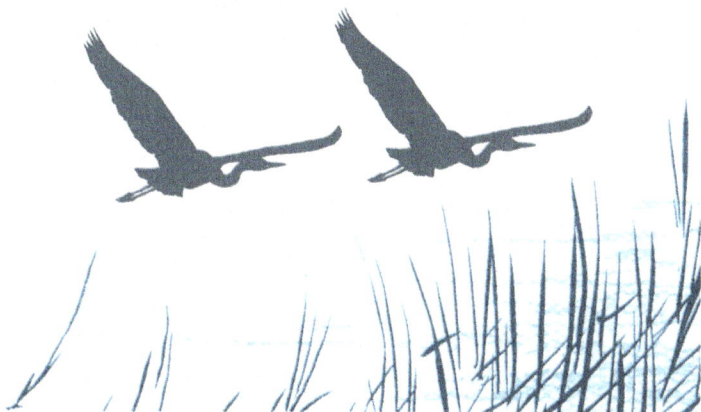

This brings us to the most reflective chapter in this book. Looking back and forward in time, where am I on this journey seven months after Gene's passing? Although I miss her greatly, I am at peace, and have accepted this as part of a larger plan. I know that I did everything possible to avert this outcome, and carry no guilt forward about not having done enough. Nor am I depressed. It is time for a new chapter. I talk to her every day, and we are still together in spirit. But there is more to do here before we mix our ashes and rest full-time!

My recent attendance in the Presbyterian Church, especially with its class on Emotionally Healthy Spirituality, has been helpful in getting to this place. With Gene's urging and permission, as expressed to me so many times over the last five years, I am open to a second love relationship. Situational loneliness has been my biggest problem in recent months, especially loss of feminine companionship and everyday conversation in a caring relationship. As for a second lover in the twilight of life, the poet Mark Strand has this to say in his book *The Late Hour*:[2]

> *Even this late it happens;*
> *The coming of love, the coming of light . . .*
> *Even this late the bones of the body shine*
> *And tomorrow's dust flares into breath.*

I have tried to slow down and become more contemplative. As Ann Voskamp says in her beautiful book, *One Thousand Gifts: A Dare to Live Fully Right Where You Are*, "Hurry always empties the soul." And further:

> *Time is a relentless river. It rages on, a respecter of no one. And this, this is the only way to slow time: When I enter time's swift current, enter into the current moment with the weight of all my attention, I slow the torrent with the weight of me all here. I can slow the torrent by being all here. I only live the full life when I live fully in the moment.*[3]

It's interesting how that ties to a dream that I had recently:

> *I was in a boat headed downstream, then found myself in the river without a life preserver; got to shore; there was Gene, with her favorite red jacket on; big kiss, then back to the river feeling happy.*

My eternal gratitude to Gene for her support, love and putting up with me over all these years. Despite the relentless progression of Alzheimer's, she triumphed by retaining her independent personhood, grace and dignity. You beat it, love, and I salute you!

Whatever the future brings, our souls are together. And they have grown. As Jerry Sittser observes in his book *A Grace Disguised: How the Soul Grows Through Loss*:

> *The soul is elastic, like a balloon. It can grow larger through suffering. Loss can enlarge its capacity for anger, depression, despair, and anguish, all natural and legitimate emotions whenever we experience loss. Once enlarged, the soul is also capable of experiencing greater joy, strength, peace and love.*[4]

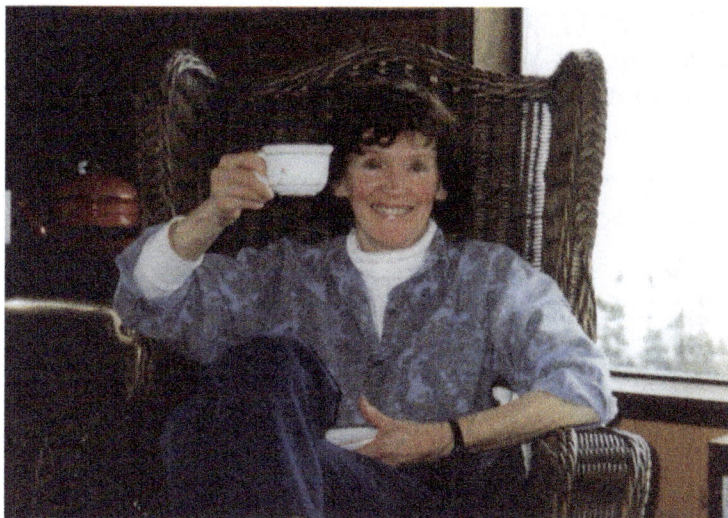

I have always been inspired by these words in John Denver's *The Eagle and the Hawk*:

Come dance with the west wind and touch on the mountain tops
Sail out over the canyons and up to the stars
And reach for the heavens and hope for the future
And all that we can be and not what we are.

Whatever the future brings, our souls will stay together, Gene's and mine, as we continue our journey in the fullness of time—our uninterrupted dance of life. The power of souls is limitless as they explore the mystery of it all. As philosopher Michael Grosso concludes in his book *Soulmaking: Uncommon Paths to Self-Understanding*:

We are more than we think we are, with more depth and expanse of being, more continuity with the past and outreach toward the future. The life of soul, then, is a life of adventure, for it involves exploring the unknown.[5]

So Gene and I, as souls together, continue our walk, hand-in-hand (if souls have hands!) with just one footprint in the sands of time.

APPENDIX I

Resources and Suggested Reading

ON ALZHEIMER'S DISEASE

National Alzheimer's Association. (www.alz.org)

As the world's leading voluntary health organization involved in Alzheimer's care, support and research, this not-for-profit organization is an essential resource for patients and caregivers. Established in 1980, it has chapters all over the country, offering many services related to description of the disease, its stages, course and treatment.

Also available is an extensive list of state and city affiliates that can provide support groups in your neighborhood. Its latest report, *Alzheimer's Disease Facts and Figures 2012,* can be downloaded from its web site. The Alzheimer's Association also has a shop that can direct you to DVDs, CDs and board games with helpful ideas about dealing with each stage of the disease.

> National Alzheimer's Association
> 225 N. Michigan Avenue
> Chicago, Illinois 60601
> 24/7 Helpline 1-800-272-3900

Amen Clinics, Inc (ACI). (www.amenclinics.com).

Established in 1989 by Daniel G. Amen, M.D., these clinics specialize in brain health and diseases. It now has four centers around the country and can be contacted at 1-888-564-2700. Useful resources include the 2012 book, *Use Your Brain to Change Your Age.* Crown Archetype, New York, 2012, with companion DVD and other DVDs: *High Performance Brains* and *Live Longer with the Brain Doctor's Wife Cookbook* by Tana Amen. Questionnaires are available for memory screening and risk assessment for Alzheimer's.

ON CAREGIVING

Nancy Mace and Peter Rabins. *The 36-Hour Day: A Family Guide to Caring for Persons with Alzheimer's Disease, Related Dementing Illnesses, and Memory Loss in Later Life.* This is the classic book in this field, issued by the Johns Hopkins University Press, with regular updated editions since it was first published in 1981.

These web sites can be useful in specific areas:

www.alz.org/stresscheck/ (to check how you are doing with loneliness and stress)

www.wellspouse.org/ (support for caregivers through the Well Spouse Association)

www.caregiver.org (Newsletter, shared personal stories and discussion groups through the Family Caregiver Alliance)

www.aarp.org/family/caregiving (housing and mobility, grandparenting, love and relationships, life after loss, on-line communities)

www.caregiver.com (how to make meal times easier for caregivers)

www.rosalynncarter.org/ (evidence-based pod casts and links to Medicare resources)

ON GRIEVING

CareNotes. Helpful notes on bereavement. www.carenotes.com (1-800-325-2511)

Alix Kates Shulman. *To Love What Is.* Farrar, Straus and Giroux, New York, 2008.

Alla Renee Bozarth. *Life Is Goodbye Life Is Hello.* Hazelden, Center City, MN, 1986.

ON THE SPIRITUAL JOURNEY

Jerry Sittser. *A Grace Disguised: How the Soul Grows Through Loss.* Zondervan, Grand Rapids, MI, 2005.

Ann Voskamp. *One Thousand Gifts: A Dare to Live Fully Right Where You Are.* Zondervan, Grand Rapids, MI, 2010.

Peter Scazzero. *Emotionally Healthy Spirituality: Unleash a Revolution in Your Life in Christ.* Thomas Nelson, Inc., Nashville, TN, 2006.

Joseph Campbell. *The Power of Myth* with Bill Moyers. Anchor Books, New York, 1988.

Dianne Arcangel. *Afterlife Encounters: Ordinary People, Extraordinary Experiences.* Hampton Roads Publishing Company, Inc., Charlottsville, VA, 2005.

Michael Grosso. *Soulmaking: Uncommon Paths to Self-Understanding.* Hampton Roads Publishing Company, Inc., Charlottsville, VA, 1997.

Notes

Chapter 4: City Life and Full-time Teaching

1. Poem by Jenny Joseph. In Sandra Martz (editor) *When I Am an Old Woman I Shall Wear Purple*. Papier Mache Press. Watsonville, CA, 1987.
2. Hermine Hilton. *50 Ways to a Better Memory*. Publications International, Ltd, 1994, p. 23.

Chapter 6: The Onset of Alzheimer's

1. J E. Brody. When lapses are not just signs of aging. *New York Times*, September 6, 2011: D7.
2. Aaron Alterra. *The Caregiver: A Life with Alzheimer's*. Steerforth Press, South Royalton, VT, 1999.
3. Daniel L. Schacter. *The Seven Sins of Memory: How the Mind Forgets and Remembers*. Houghton Mifflin Company, Boston, 2001, p. 61.
4. Julian Whitaker, *The Memory Solution*. Avery Publishing Group, New York, 1999.

Chapter 12: Moving to Town

1. Barry Peterson. *Jan's Story: Love Lost to the Long Goodbye of Alzheimer's*. Behler Publications, Lake Forest, CA 2010.

Chapter 16: An Empty House

1. W. Dewi Rees. The hallucinations of widowhood. *British Medical Journal*, pp. 37-41, October 2, 1971.

Chapter 18: Bereavement

1. Jerry Sittser. *A Grace Disguised: How the Soul Grows Through Loss.* Zondervan, Grand Rapids, MI, 2004, p. 17.
2. Ibid, p. 73.
3. C. S. Lewis. *A Grief Observed.* Harper Collins Publishers, New York, 1961, p. 50.

Chapter 19: What I Have Learned

1. From Joseph Campbell. *The Power of Myth* with Bill Moyers, Doubleday, New York, 1988, p. 231.
2. Shirley Wang. France seeks new ways to manage Alzheimer's care. *Wall Street Journal*, Oct. 18, 2012: A11
3. Aaron Alterra. *The Caregiver.* Steerforth Press, South Royalton, MI, 1999, pp 203-4.
4. Dianne Arcangel. *Afterlife Encounters: Ordinary People, Extraordinary Experiences.* Hampton Roads Publishing Company, Inc. Charlottsville, VA, 2005.

Chapter 20: Souls Walking On

1. Jerry Sittser. *A Grace Disguised: How the Soul Grows Through Loss.* Zondervan, Grand Rapids, MI, 2004, p. 199.
2. Mark Strand, poet and author of *The Late Hour,* as quoted by Gail Sheehy in her book *Understanding Men's Passages,* Ballantine Books, New York, 1999, p. 260

3. Voskamp, A. *One Thousand Gifts: A Dare to Live Fully Right Where You Are*. Zondervan, Grand Rapids, MI, 2010, p. 68.
4. Ibid # 1, p. 48.
5. Michael Grosso. *Soulmaking: Uncommon Paths to Self-Understanding*. Hampton Roads Publishing Company, Inc. Charlottsville, VA, 1997, p. 199.

Discussion Questions

General

1. If you are faced with the care of your spouse or family member with Alzheimer's, what new life plan would you consider for yourself and your family?

2. How would you have handled the decision to continue care at home in your own community vs. moving to another community and facility?

3. If you had to move to care for a family member with Alzheimer's, where would you go, and how would the move impact your own life?

4. Would you have taken a different approach to the timing and decision to abandon "curative" care for comfort care?

5. In what ways does this story resonate with you and your family's history?

6. If you have had a family member develop Alzheimer's, how old were they at its onset, how was their course, and what does that mean for you and your family?

7. What narrative in your own, and your spouse's life, would you want to be honored by your spouse and his/her physicians in choosing options for care of Alzheimer's?

8. Do you have long-term care insurance, and if so, how good would its coverage be for care of Alzheimer's? Would you be able to afford care for a family member with Alzheimer's?

9. Given what you now know about Gene's and John's lives together, why do you think that John ended up deciding to write this book?

Caregiving and Coping

1. Do you have family, friends and a supportive community if you have to deal with the care of a family member with Alzheimer's?

2. If you become the primary caregiver of your spouse with Alzheimer's, how would you reach out to family, friends and the community?

3. If you were faced with the challenge of your spouse developing Alzheimer's disease, at what points do you feel you would no longer be able to serve as the primary caregiver at home?

4. Would you have arranged for caregivers earlier than John did, and if so, in what way?

5. If your spouse develops Alzheimer's, would you be able to talk to him/her about how to proceed?

6. How would you cope with your spouse's increasing dependence on you as the primary caregiver, including changing moods and intermittent anger?

7. If you become the primary caregiver for your spouse with Alzheimer's, how would you protect yourself, and how would you arrange for your own respite care?

8. Do you have an Advance Directive and Physician Orders for Life-Sustaining Treatment (POLST) (p. 187)? If not, why not?

Bereavement and the Future

1. If you have to face the loss of your spouse after a long and happy marriage, and knowing that everyone grieves in a different way, how do you think that you would respond?

2. What opportunities would you see for the future of your own life?

3. Are there spiritual resources you would call upon?